Healthy Eating for Men

Get Back in Shape, Prevent Health problems, Lose Weight and Stay Fit at Any Age

Michael Smith

© **Copyright 2020 - All rights reserved.**

The content contained within this book may not be reproduced, duplicated or transmitted without direct written permission from the author or the publisher.
Under no circumstances will any blame or legal responsibility be held against the publisher, or author, for any damages, reparation, or monetary loss due to the information contained within this book, either directly or indirectly.
Legal Notice:
This book is copyright protected. It is only for personal use. You cannot amend, distribute, sell, use, quote or paraphrase any part, or the content within this book, without the consent of the author or publisher.
Disclaimer Notice:
Please note the information contained within this document is for educational and entertainment purposes only. All effort has been executed to present accurate, up to date, reliable, complete information. No warranties of any kind are declared or implied. Readers acknowledge that the author is not engaged in the rendering of legal, financial, medical or professional advice. The content within this book has been derived from various sources. Please consult a licensed professional before attempting any techniques outlined in this book.
By reading this document, the reader agrees that under no circumstances is the author responsible for any losses, direct or indirect, that are incurred as a result of the use of the information contained within this document, including, but not limited to, errors, omissions, or inaccuracies.

Table of Contents

TABLE OF CONTENTS 3

INTRODUCTION 6

YOU ARE NOT ALONE 6
IT'S ALL ABOUT NUTRITION AND LIFESTYLE 7
YOU CAN DO THIS 10
YOUR PERSONAL PLAN FOR A HEALTHY DIET AND LIFESTYLE 12

CHAPTER 1: WITH MATURITY, THESE PROBLEMS CAN SNEAK UP ON YOU 15

HOW ARE YOU FEELING? 15
THE BIGGEST RISK 17
Heart Disease 17
Cardiovascular Risk Factors 17
Some Examples 24
How to Prevent Heart Disease 26
THE OTHER RISKS 27
Overall Guidelines For Mature Men 31
See Your Healthcare Provider 36

CHAPTER 2: CAN HEALTHY EATING TURN YOUR HEALTH AROUND? 39

THEMES AND PRINCIPLES 39
THE RESPECTED RESOURCES 41
The 80:20 Principle 42
The China Study 49
Benefits of a Healthy Diet 51
Harvard School of Public Health 53

CHAPTER 3: WHAT SHOULD I EAT 61

DIETARY RECOMMENDATIONS BY FOOD GROUP 62
Recommended Carbohydrates 64
Recommended Plant-Based Proteins 69

3

Recommended Meat Proteins.. *73*
Meat Protein Cautions.. *74*
Recommended Fats and Oils *76*

CHAPTER 4: WHAT SHOULD I DRINK....................................... 81

WATER WE NEED 82
SUGAR IN BEVERAGES...84
More Than You Realize *84*
NUTRITIOUS BEVERAGES 88
Apple Cider Vinegar *88*
Coffee is Approved.. *90*
ALCOHOL: FACTS AND FICTIONS..97
Alcohol in Moderation *97*
Alcohol: The Downsides *100*

CHAPTER 5: MICRONUTRIENTS AND SUPPLEMENTS 105

DOES A MATURE MAN NEED SUPPLEMENTS? 105
Are Supplements Necessary? *107*
Fortified Foods *108*
Playing It Safe with Supplements *109*
How Much Do You Need? *111*
Collagen Supplements *114*
Testosterone..*118*

CHAPTER 6: HEALTHY EATING IN PRACTICE...................... 122

YOUR INDIVIDUAL DIET 123
Guidelines, Not Conformity..*124*
Food Sensitivities...*125*
The Recommended Mediterranean Diet *128*
Planning for Special Dietary Goals..*131*
Sticking With Your Healthy Diet...*135*
Intermittent Fasting *138*
7-Day Meal Plan..*141*

CHAPTER 7: LIFESTYLE TIPS FOR MAXIMUM SUCCESS ... 145

THE BENEFITS OF EXERCISE... 145
MEDITATION AND MINDFULNESS... 153
MENTAL STIMULATION AND SOCIAL INTERACTION 157

THE BENEFITS OF SLEEP 159
   Sleep and Your Immune System 161

CHAPTER 8: EASY AND DELICIOUS RECIPES FOR YOUR OPTIMAL HEALTH 163

BREAKFAST RECIPES 164
   Breakfast Recipe #1 - Spicy Apple Oatmeal with Egg 164
   Breakfast Recipe #2 - Homemade Hot Muesli 167
   Breakfast Recipe #3 - Overnight Oat Muesli 169
   Breakfast Recipe #4 - Hearty Turkey Bacon and Eggs 171
LUNCH RECIPES 174
   Lunch Recipe #5 - Chickpeas, Greens Salad & Tuna .. 174
   Lunch Recipe # 6 - Grilled Salmon with Brown Rice . 177
   Lunch Recipe #7 - Greek Chicken Salad 180
   Lunch Recipe #8 - Steamed Mussels with Quinoa 183
   Lunch Recipe #9 - Vegetarian Split Pea Soup 186
   Lunch Recipe # 10 - Fast Tuna Over Whole Grain Pasta 189
   Lunch Recipe #11 - Split Pea Soup (with meat) 192
DINNER RECIPES 194
   Dinner Recipe #12 - Steamed Fish with Potatoes and Tomatoes 194
   Dinner Recipe #13 - Italian Meatballs and Spaghetti 198
   Dinner Recipe #14 - Steamed Shrimp with Tomatoes and Pasta 202
   Dinner Recipe #15 - Chicken Scaloppine Marsala Sauté with Polenta 205
   Dinner Recipe #16 - Mediterranean Fish Stew 208
   Dinner Recipe #17 - Mediterranean Grilled Chicken over Spinach 211
   Dinner Recipe #18 - Steamed Seafood Mix with Tomatoes and Pasta 214

CONCLUSION 216

YOUR FREE GIFT 219

REFERENCES 220

Introduction

You Are Not Alone

If you are a mature man, and facing health and wellbeing concerns, you are certainly not alone. All men are subject to the changes and challenges that come with reaching midlife years, and beyond. You have a choice: to surrender to the inevitable signs and symptoms of aging or to take the alternative path of defending yourself against deterioration, disability and loss of energy and spirit. If you are ready to adopt a proactive lifestyle that really works, and is backed by science and experience, this is the only guide you will need.

What are the issues that concern you?

> Do you anticipate physical and emotional problems that come after reaching middle age, and think that your health is at risk with the diseases and conditions of aging?

> Do you think your dietary practices are not optimal for your health, and that you should be paying more attention to your nutrition? Is your immune system optimal?

> Are you remembering days gone by when you kept in shape, and are wondering if it's

possible to bring back the energy and vitality you feel that you've lost?

Do worries and anxieties keep you up at night, preventing restful sleep and keeping you on edge? Are you tenser, and subject to bouts of depression?

It's not too late to turn around what you thought were the inevitable downturns of health and fitness—both physical and mental. Starting today, you can begin to reverse the signs of aging, potentially increasing your longevity, and keeping you healthier and happier longer.

It s All About Nutrition and Lifestyle

Your health involves much more than simply trying to cope with being middle age; it requires a personal lifestyle reinvention to restore lost energy, become healthier, and feel better than you have in years. Will the adoption of a new lifestyle of good nutrition, weight management and fitness help you live longer? As the adage goes, it may *add more years to your life*, and it will definitely *put more life into your years*.

Reaching middle-age is a milestone to be proud of, but it's also a time to evaluate how you're doing, and how it's going. Whether you're just hitting 40, or have gone beyond the half-century mark, the goal is to be in the best health and best shape you can be. But it's important to recognize and acknowledge that you've changed, and will continue to change as the years inevitably accumulate. Hormone levels, including testosterone, are slowly but steadily lowering, muscle mass is reducing, and fat cells are replacing muscle. Your shape is changing, and that lower gut is making its presence known. Goodbye six-pack abs; hello pot belly. Your immune system may not be optimal; either not as good at detecting and dispatching pathogens, or overreacting and causing chronic inflammation.

Of all the serious conditions you may be thinking about is your cardiovascular health. Most mature men may be making their first visit to a cardiologist, getting a cholesterol reading learning about HDL (good) cholesterol and LDL (bad) cholesterol. You are probably aware that diet and exercise, weight management, and cessation of smoking are actions that are under your control.

You can have science and research on your side, to separate fact from fiction, and get you on the right track to optimal health, energy, strength and fitness. I recently reached my 50th birthday, and I began trying all the hyped-up shortcuts, and exaggerated promises, until I got back to the basics of solid research, scientific facts, and quantitative, clinical trials, reported by the Cleveland Clinic, Johns Hopkins Medical Center, the Mayo Clinic, the Harvard Medical Review, Scientific American, and other respected authorities. I began looking for answers in books like "Eat, Drink, and Be Healthy," "Forks Over Knives," and "Bigger, Leaner, Stronger". I learned how important our digestive system is in affecting the responses and effectiveness of our immune system in protecting us from diseases.

Getting to this point took a lot of time and testing. Cutting back on meat, upping the protein, lowering the carbohydrates, reducing sugar, eliminating sugar, celebrity diets, ketogenic diets, reduced fats, regional diets from places where people live longer, paleo diets (in case our Homo sapiens ancestors knew some secrets). I studied and practiced intermittent fasting, like 16:8, where you can eat during 8 hours and then fast for 16 hours. I've tried eating whole grains (instead of refined) and even started eating whole grain sourdough bread. I tried eliminating gluten and took supplements to raise my fiber intake. In case I had any food allergies, I tried the new FODMAP diet which eliminates foods that ferment incorrectly in your gut. (Did you know that trillions of bacteria live in your digestive system, and most of them are beneficial? The right diet keeps this microbiome in balance and at full effectiveness).

Now you can benefit from my years of studying and testing, because I've combined all of this valid research with my own positive experience to share with you, and to create a step-by-step, realistic, achievable roadmap to help you prevent age-related health problems, feel great, and get much more out of life.

You Can Do This

Are you concerned that adopting a healthy lifestyle built around nutritious dietary and lifestyle practices is difficult? Rest assured, it is easier than you think. Will this mean giving up all the foods and beverages you like, and having to limit your diet to bland and boring foods? Not at all, and you will be pleasantly surprised to discover new foods and eating practices that you can embrace with enthusiasm. You are in the right place to find facts separated from fiction, and healthy, effective diets instead of ineffective fad diets.

Let me share my own personal experience, since I've been through what you are facing. I approached middle age with the priorities of building a career and raising a family. I had been active when I was young, with sports, always in motion, with lots of energy. I ate what I wanted, as much as I wanted, whenever I wanted it, and never thought about weight management or nutrition. I was young, strong, moving up. But one day, not too long ago, I looked in the mirror, and said to myself, "Hey, who is that guy"? I had entered a new age group, and with it, I discovered an expanding gut, a softer set of muscles, greater susceptibility to illness, and a feeling that I "didn't have it" anymore. I had a choice then, as you have now: give in to aging, or look it in the eye, and say, "No way."

Now I'm that I'm 50, my life has evolved, as your life surely is evolving now. The ladder-climbing career mindset is less of a priority, and options for alternative lifestyles are starting to appear. If you raised a family, as I did, the kids grow up, and you are finding that you're not needed by them anymore, and you have more personal time available. But with the slowing down, you may not have the energy and spirit to take advantage of that time. Do you find yourself getting soft, discovering a bigger waistline, having less get-up-and-go? Is this inevitable, or could your lifestyle have something to do with it? Have you given up on the opportunities for romance, whether it's with a long time wife or partner, or with someone new?

It's entirely up to you. It's your choice to seize the moment and regain what has been slowly slipping away. Are you ready to change your lifestyle to one of health and wellbeing? You know the answer. You can do this.

Your Personal Plan for a Healthy Diet and Lifestyle

We'll start by identifying the problems that can sneak up when you're a man who has reached the midlife mark. If you continue down the path of ignoring the need for good nutrition and dietary practices, you may be confronted by impactful problems and conditions you're aware of, and some that you don't realize may be waiting, just down the road. Next, we'll get right down to where most of the problems are caused, and where they can be reversed or prevented. Yes, I'm talking about nutrition, which has influence over your health more than all other factors combined.

This leads to what you should eat. We'll look at the popular dietary option, weigh their pros and cons, and then focus on the one diet that is universally respected as the most healthful, while also being great tasting, filling, and satisfying. Your ideal, health-giving diet also includes beverages, and we'll discuss what to drink, what not to drink. and why. Don't worry, you'll have plenty of good options to choose from.

What about dietary supplements and micronutrients? Are they necessary? Do they work? What does the Food and Drug Administration (FDA) have to say about these supplements? You'll come away understanding how to distinguish the necessary, effective supplements from all those that overpromise and make unsubstantiated claims.

Now you will be ready to consider your options and make intelligent, informed choices about what to eat and drink, how to eat in moderation without counting calories, and how to step up to the oven and prepare the recipes that will get you started and well underway. No need to become a chef, but depending on your time available, you can impart your own personal touch to some, or all, of your meals. Nutritious, delicious meals can be simple, with minimal preparation. There's a world of creative invention waiting for you in the kitchen.

We'll wrap up with the lifestyle improvements that do not involve diet and nutrition, by explaining the need for physical and mental activity, including cardiovascular, resistance and flexibility exercise, getting a good night's sleep, managing stress, anxiety, and depression, and other influences on your health and longevity. We'll complete this section with some of the newest techniques to get into shape, stay calm and in control, sleep better, and stay relaxed; all of which will contribute to optimizing your health and wellbeing.

If you want to read more, especially to follow up with the medical and professional articles that contributed to this book, many of which are cited in the text, turn to the **References** section at the end of the book: You'll find every source listed alphabetically by author, and with the article title and a hyperlink that will take you there with a click.

I'm excited to share with you what I've learned and benefitted from, and hope you achieve the same improvements in health, attitude and outlook. Okay, let's get started.

Michael Smith,

Boca Raton, Florida, 2020

Chapter 1: With Maturity, These Problems Can Sneak Up on You

If you are a man who has reached the good age of midlife and continues with the careless nutritional and lifestyle habits of your younger years, and you do nothing to recognize the changes that reaching this level of maturity inevitably brings, you risk being susceptible to age and gender-related health problems. How well you live, and how long you live, are potentially under your control. Many of the conditions and illnesses that accompany your maturity can be prevented or at least slowed and diminished in their onset. Early prevention is the preferable option, so let's see how to get a jump on what's coming.

How Are You Feeling?

Perhaps you've made it this far without too many medical and health issues. Sure, you've had your share of colds, maybe a flu or two, aches and pains, some indigestion, a few sports injuries that have healed, but not the big ones. As far as you know, your heart seems to be in good shape, and nothing serious is affecting you. Or is it?

Behind the curtain, if you are middle-aged man things are changing, and it's better to know what might be coming, than let a condition or reduced ability, or a disease creep up and blindside you. Your best defense is a strong offense, which means you will be anticipating the problems, and heading them off before they manifest themselves.

In this chapter, we're going to lift the curtain and see what conditions may be coming your way, and take a first look at what to do about it. In subsequent chapters we will address the major lifestyle changes you will want to be making to be in the best state of health you can be. Let's get started.

The Biggest Risk

Heart Disease

We'll begin with the big one. Sure, sore knees and aching joints and low sex drive are concerns, and we'll get into those, but existential threats come first. One in two—52% of all middle-age men—will develop heart disease at some point, according to the Centers for Disease Control (CDC), and 50% of the men who will die from heart disease don't even know they have it, due to a lack of symptoms. A mature man may feel great, eat responsibly, keep in shape, yet things may be going on that can have serious implications down the road. Doctors at Northwestern University and numerous other medical institutions found that the onset of heart disease depends on certain "risk factors." The probability of developing heart disease is 69% for men with two or more risk factors by age 50, but only 9% for men without risk factors at that age.

Cardiovascular Risk Factors

Risk factors for heart disease were initially identified by the *Framingham Heart Study*, the longest-running, large scale study of heart disease. The study began in 1948 and is now in its fourth generation of participants.

Importantly, the same precautionary directions for heart disease are applicable to virtually all other diseases and conditions that we maturing men have to watch out for, including type 2 diabetes, obesity, high blood sugar, and even cancer and cognitive disorders.

These are the most commonly cited cardiovascular risk factors from the Framingham Heart Study, according to Donald M. Lloyd-Jones, MD, ScM, who part of the medical team responsible for the lifetime risk assessment:

> **Age:** Being a middle-aged man is the first level of concern; reaching age 65 is the next level. Age, by itself, does not cause problems, but is a marker of a man's coming to an age of vulnerability.
>
>> A close friend is a former marathon runner; he kept in shape, followed what he thought was a healthy diet, didn't smoke, and yet, in his mid-60s, my friend was diagnosed with exercise-induced angina (chest pain), due to a buildup of plaque in his coronary arteries. It's under good control now, but had this been diagnosed earlier, when he reached

age 55, the buildup could have been stopped much sooner.

Family history: If a parent had a heart attack before age 50, you may have a risk of a congenital, or inherited risk of early heart disease. Genetics can play an influential role in causing heart disease, in spite of the normal precautions. If your family history points to a risk of early-onset heart disease, it is important to be under the care of a cardiologist. A genetic propensity towards the following risk factors may be unavoidable, but with good precautionary care, the symptoms may be limited or even eliminated.

Cholesterol: This fatty, waxy substance is produced in the liver, and plays an important role in various functions, but one form, low-density lipoprotein (LDL), can adhere to artery walls and cause a buildup of plaque, which can reduce blood flow, especially to the coronary arteries that bring oxygen to the heart. LDL is called 'bad 'cholesterol, while high-density lipoprotein (HDL), or 'good 'cholesterol is believed to be beneficial, by carrying away LDL cholesterol before it can harden into plaque.

Triglycerides: This is a yellowish fat that accumulates in the blood when there is too much fat in the diet, especially saturated fat found in red meat, butter, and some cheeses. High triglycerides are an indication that there is an excess of fat being stored in the body, and may contribute to heart disease.

High Blood Pressure: Also called hypertension, high blood pressure is now designated as pressure readings of 140/80, or higher. The first number, the systolic pressure, is a measurement of pressure in the arteries when the heartbeats, or pumps, and the second, number, diastolic, is the pressure between beats. The primary risk of high blood pressure is stroke (either a blockage in a brain artery or a burst brain artery). Lifestyle changes, including diet and exercise, and limiting salt (sodium) in the diet, can help lower blood pressure, but medication may be necessary in many cases. High blood pressure should not be ignored.

Obesity: Becoming overweight is often a gradual process of gaining 1-2 pounds per year. Over a period of 25 years, that can add up to 50 extra pounds. But as explained in "The Obesity Code: Unlocking the Secrets of

Weight Loss" (Fung, J. 2016), research has shown that weight management is not about counting calories, but more a matter of hormonal activity. He says that the traditional view of obesity as a caloric imbalance did not add up when the evidence is reviewed. Doctors have been prescribing calorie reduction for the past 50 years, with few positive results, Dr. Fung summarizes. He felt that something else was needed for effective weight management, especially to prevent, or reduce, type 2 diabetes. His studies demonstrated that insulin levels are pivotal in weight gain, and high blood insulin is the most influential factor, far more than calories, in causing weight gain, and in defeating efforts to lose weight.

While caloric reduction may trigger short-term losses, the results don't last because cutting calories does not deal with the underlying issue, which is hormonal imbalances that accrue from years of unhealthy diets, leading to elevated levels of the hormone insulin. So weight loss can't be addressed by lowering calories or by exercise; it can only be resolved by bringing insulin levels back into balance.

Inactivity: A healthy heart is an active heart. The evolution of our species, Homo sapiens, and our predecessor species, is based on hundreds of thousands of years, during which time, people were in continuous physical movement. Up until late in the 19th century, our ancestors were hunter/gatherers, and later, into the 20th century, farmers and laborers. There was no traveling by cars, buses, trains, and airplanes; no sitting at desks and tables all day, and on a sofa all evening. We evolved as movers and shakers, always up and about, physically busy. That is who we were, and that is who we still are.

Today, when we are sedentary, our cardiovascular system becomes lazy, and the negative effects of improper diets are exacerbated. Genetic tendencies to accumulate plaque, or to retain fat and become obese, are not stopped or slowed. We'll give you good direction on how to get in shape and stay in shape in chapter 8, lifestyle tips for maximum success.

Smoking: If you are not a smoker, that's great; don't start. As you will see in the following overall guidelines, smoking is perhaps the most dangerous of all the risk factors, and not just for preventing heart disease.

If you have tried to stop smoking, and nothing has worked, follow the recommendations of the many satisfied readers of "Allen Carr's Easy Way to Stop Smoking." (Carr, A, 2011). Over 20 million copies have been sold, which is more than all other books for quitting smoking combined. It's been the top seller in nine European countries. The latest edition, available at Amazon, is the U.S. version. It's a simple, easy-to-follow, drug-free process that millions of smokers, including more than a few of my own associates, have found works for them,

Alcohol. If you are not a drinker, most doctors recommend you don't start. But if you are a moderate drinker, the medical community is okay with that; just don't overdo it. More about how much is enough in the guidelines, below.

Type 2 Diabetes. Also known as adult-onset diabetes, this is a disease closely associated with obesity. As reported in the

University of California, San Francisco's *Diabetes Education Online* (2020), the pancreas produces and normally releases insulin, which controls the level of glucose, or sugar, in the blood. Diabetics do not have sufficient insulin to control sugar levels. Type 2 diabetes is considered a risk factor for cardiovascular disease, and is often associated with obesity. The onset of diabetes can be slowed or prevented by maintaining normal body weight and following a healthy, nutritious diet.

Some of these risk factors are outside your control, notably your family history and your genetic profile, but most other risk factors are very much influenced by your lifestyle decisions. You decide what and how much you eat, how much you weigh, whether you smoke, how much alcohol you consume, whether you exercise regularly. You also have the ability to help manage serum cholesterol levels and blood pressure.

Some Examples

Generally, there is no single risk factor that causes heart disease, but rather the cumulative effect of several.

> For example, a person may have a genetic predisposition to high LDL (bad) cholesterol, which causes the buildup of plaque in the coronary arteries that supply the heart with oxygen. Added to that, the person smokes, is overweight, and is sedentary, meaning physically inactive.

The person we've just described has a profile of someone likely to suffer a heart attack, perhaps not immediately, but within a reasonable number of years. The risk increases once age 65 is reached, but by then, quite a bit of damage is done, with partially blocked coronary arteries, or of arteries in the legs, a condition called Peripheral Artery Disease (PAD). The blockages can impede the flow of oxygen-given blood to the heart, and cause permanent damage to the myocardium, the heart muscle. Eventually, a piece of the plaque can detach, and block the blood flow in the coronary artery completely, causing a coronary occlusion, a classic heart attack.

> Another person may have a genetic tendency to hypertension or high blood pressure. In this case, a diet with too much salt (sodium) keeps the blood pressure high (above 140/80). Depending on other factors, this person has increased susceptibility to a stroke—either a blocked artery in the brain,

caused by a clot, or a burst artery in the brain, as the result of a weakening of the artery wall by years of high blood pressure.

How to Prevent Heart Disease

Men who have reached the midlife mark are advised to follow a two-prong strategy to optimize their cardiovascular health and slow or stop the onset and progression of heart disease:

1. **See a cardiologist.** Have your cardiovascular health checked regularly, and follow your doctor's advice. In subsequent chapters, we'll get into all of the diet and lifestyle changes you can take to reduce the risk of heart disease, but be open to medications your doctor may recommend to further reduce the risk. For example, as the pharmaceutical company says, credibly, "When diet and exercise are not enough," you may be prescribed an LDL cholesterol-lowering drug called a statin. The best known is Lipitor, generic name atorvastatin. You may also be instructed to take a small 'baby 'aspirin every night, which reduces the 'stickiness 'of blood and helps prevent clots that can cause a heart attack or a stroke.

2. **Manage your lifestyle**. Take charge of your heart through diet, exercise and lifestyle changes that can reduce the risk factors and keep you healthier, longer. Many other health concerns are addressed by these same changes. Starting in the next chapter, we'll get into all aspects of diet, recipes, and all the other lifestyle recommendations, but for now, use the information in this section to get a first grounding in the principles.

The Other Risks

Mature, middle-aged men begin to become concerned about loss of strength, vitality, sex drive, and other symbols of masculinity. We also become aware of stiffness in the joints, reduced flexibility, and a bit of slowing down. These conditions are a natural function of aging, but can be mediated by good nutrition in most cases. But there are also conditions that may require hormonal adjustments or medical care. Here are the most common concerns among mature men:

Testosterone, the male hormone produced in the testicles begins to decline after midlife. The American Urological Association says that 20% of men over 60 have low levels of testosterone, and that rises to 30% after 70 (*Healthline*, 2019). Do you need to worry? It's a good idea to have your testosterone level checked every five years after age 50, and don't be concerned with gradual lowering; it's a normal part of aging. If levels remain within the normal range, there's no need for supplements.

But if you have some symptoms, which Ryan Wallace and Kathleen Yoder cite in *Healthline* (2019), which may include reduced sex drive, erectile dysfunction, fatigue, loss of energy, reduced muscle mass, or depression and mood changes, it could be a sign that your doctor may need to prescribe a form of hormone replacement therapy. But first, get tested, since these symptoms can be due to other causes.

Osteoporosis. This condition causes bones to become porous, brittle, and more susceptible to breaking. The right nutrients, including calcium, can strengthen your bones to avoid breaking, by preventing osteoporosis, which occurs with greater frequency when men age. According to *WebMD* (2020), you may become aware of more frequent backaches, stooped posture and loss of height, or experience breakage in wrist or hands. If your diet includes dairy products, you probably get enough calcium, but if a bone density test shows that you do have osteoporosis, your doctor may prescribe medication to firm things up.

Collagen. Mature men need to be aware of their need for collagen, which is the most abundant protein that we have. Collagen production begins to diminish starting at age 21. By the age of 40, the loss is typically 1% per year and at age of 50 men have about -10% less collagen production.

Kerri-Ann Jennings, RN (Healthline, 2020), says that collagen is essential in helping in the construction of cells, tissue, organs, and muscles, as well as being the 'glue 'that helps hold protein molecules together. Vitamin C helps rebuild collagen, along with the amino acids proline and glycine, which are found in eggs, dairy, and meats. Nuts and seeds are good sources of the mineral copper, which also contributes to collagen regeneration.

Acid Reflux. This occurs when the hydrochloric acid in your gut leaks upwards into your esophagus and causes a burning sensation. If it occurs infrequently, it's just indigestion, and a simple antacid, like Tums or Rolaids can get rid of the symptoms quickly. But if it occurs more frequently, it can become gastroesophageal reflux disease (GERD), and lead to damage to the esophagus. As reported by Markus MacGill in *Medical News Today* (2017), the American College of Gastroenterology says that more than 60 million

Americans experience acid reflux or indigestion at least once a month, and 15 million have it as often as daily, if untreated. Acid reflux-related disorders are the leading cause of visits to the hospital for gut distress.

In addition to avoiding certain heavy or greasy or spicy foods, and not going to sleep on a full stomach, preventative treatments are available OTC: H2 (histamine) blockers, like Pepcid, or proton-pump inhibitors (PPI) like Nexium and Prevacid. Stronger versions may be prescribed by your doctor.

Immune System Issues. Your immune system is your body's defense against infection and invading pathogens. According to *WebMD* (2020), you can boost your defenses through diet and exercise (which we'll get into later, but everything applicable to heart health also applies here). In addition, you can improve your immune health by learning to relax, stay positive, socialize and interact with people (more about this in the section on meditation and mindfulness).

Stiff Joints, Osteoarthritis, Rheumatoid Arthritis. The ends of our bones are protected by a spongy substance called cartilage. As we get into our 50's, the cartilage starts to dry out, becoming stiff and less flexible. *WebMD* (2020) reports another contributing factor: diminishing levels of synovial fluid, which normally acts as a lubricant—we make less of it as we age. These two occurrences lead to stiff, painful joints, and loss of range of motion. The recommended first line of defense is to keep moving, and it will help keep the joints loose.

Osteoarthritis occurs when the cartilage wears away, and the bone joints rub together. Rheumatoid arthritis is caused by the immune system attacking the joints, especially in the wrist and fingers. Your doctor can prescribe anti-rheumatic drugs to reduce inflammation.

Becoming a middle-aged man leaves you more vulnerable to joint injury, so take it easy, especially when lifting objects and when working out (exercise is strongly recommended for virtually all conditions, but be cognizant of not being as young as you once were).

Overall Guidelines For Mature Men

As you have seen, the need for cardiovascular health and care extends to a wide range of actions, all of which involve changes to your lifestyle; changes that affect not only heart and circulation, but to virtually every other condition that middle-aged men have to be concerned about. I've turned to the respected **Cleveland Clinic** (rated #2 medical services in America, again in 2020, by *US News & World Reports*), which lists these healthy guidelines for men over the age of 50. Don't be surprised to see the same steps, procedures, and disciplines for preventing heart disease; there is consistency in the diet and lifestyle practices that are good for health overall.

Eat a healthy diet. This tops the list of guidelines, and with good reason, since the quality of your diet can lead to *not only* improved cardiovascular health, and prevention of heart disease, but also a stronger immune system to help you fight every type of invading pathogen, trouble-free digestion, better weight control, preventing the onset of type 2 diabetes, and even help prevent certain types of cancer.

In the next chapters, we'll cover foods and beverages in detail, but in overview, Cleveland Clinic instructs us to emphasize vegetables and fruits, fish, lean meats and poultry, olive oil, nuts, whole grains, and low-fat dairy products. On the avoidance list are meats that are high in saturated fats, processed meats, trans fats. We're also advised to go easy on salt, since sodium can raise blood pressure levels. Beware, too, of added sugar and its 'empty 'calories. When we review beverages you will learn about hidden sugar in soda, and less obviously, even in sports beverages.

Maintain a healthy weight. Today in America, one-third of the adult male population is overweight, and another one-third are categorized as obese. These terms are based on the Body Mass Index (BMI), which compares height, weight, age and gender. A BMI from 18.5 to 24.9 is normal, 25 to 29.9 is overweight, and 30 and above is obese. You can easily measure your BMI online by using search terms "BMI" or "Body Mass Index." You should honestly acknowledge if you are overweight or obese, and resolve to get those extra pounds off. In subsequent chapters, you will discover how to lose weight gradually and steadily, and keep it off.

We'll review certain diets, including "The Obesity Code," written by Jason Fung, MD, and which advocates a dietary regiment specifically for those who have trouble losing weight with the usual diet and exercise routines. Dr. Fung claims that there is a "fat-burning code" in each of us, and it can be reset with intermittent fasting. Interestingly, Dr. Fung's concept is based on our evolutionary lifestyle as hunter/gatherers, when eating was more intermittent. We'll reference a fact-checked review of this diet, reported by Sumner Banks, in *DietSpotlight* (2020).

Get a good night's sleep. And do it consistently. It's time to stop thinking that you don't need a certain amount of sleep; it's been proven that our bodies, and especially our brains, need an average of eight hours of sleep every night. The CDC, in "How Much Sleep Do You Need?" (2020), recommends between 7 and 9 hours of sleep for all adults, including up to 65, but 7 to 8 hours for men over 65. During sleep, our brain reviews, sorts, files, and deletes the impressions of the previous day, just like a computer that has to be rebooted when it gets overloaded. A full night's sleep allows the brain to sweep out damaged cells and proteins. If left unchecked, these proteins can accumulate and possibly lead to Alzheimer's disease, and other forms of dementia.

We'll provide good advice on how to sleep well in a later chapter, but for now, be aware that you should go to sleep and wake up at the same time consistently, and you should not be looking at a computer or mobile phone screen for an hour before bed. Considering a nightcap? Studies show that alcohol consumed just before bedtime can interfere with REM sleep, when dreaming occurs.

Be physically active. This means regular exercise, and not allowing yourself to be sedentary. Scroll back up and review the section on inactivity. As explained in the previous section on heart health, we are designed by our evolution to be in motion, and standing, walking, bending, and climbing. Current medical protocols call for exercising at least three times a week for a weekly total of 140 minutes. Better still is to be active whenever you get the chance, and trying for walking 10,000 steps a day. We'll cover the basics of cardio and resistance exercises later on.

Do not smoke. It's more than worth the effort to stop. You read about this above, and it's something you are undoubtedly aware of. There are few things legally available that are so detrimental to your health, and completely lacking in redeeming value. Decades of scientific studies directly link tobacco to heart disease, cancer, and respiratory diseases. The nicotine and tars in tobacco have been clinically proven to not only be carcinogenic, but are also addictive, so if you smoke and are having difficulty quitting, seek professional help.

Drink alcohol in moderation. This is not to encourage non-drinkers to imbibe, but, if you drink, follow the guideline that men should limit their consumption to two drinks per day. Many studies find that moderate drinking can be beneficial, but heavy drinking can be seriously detrimental to health and longevity. So keep it to two 5 ounce glasses of wine, or two 12 ounce glasses of beer, or two 1.5 ounce servings of distilled spirits. You may have heard about an ingredient in red wine, resveratrol, and its benefits. We'll cover this in chapter 4, on what you should drink.

It's important to avoid drinking distilled spirits 'straight, 'as in tequila shots, for example. Why? Over 50, your esophagus doesn't appreciate the 'burn 'of direct contact with alcohol, and over time, straight, undiluted spirits can lead to gastroesophageal damage. Serve "on the rocks," or mixed with water or other beverages. It's safer, and you'll get more of a taste experience.

See Your Healthcare Provider

Schedule screenings and exams. When you were younger, you went to the doctor when you were sick, or perhaps for an injury. But now, men over 40 should make visits annually. It doesn't matter how you feel, because many serious illnesses and conditions are asymptomatic—they do not appear until it may be late for effective treatment. An exam by your internist or family physician will get your heart and blood pressure checked, your breathing, your vital functions, and blood tests and urine analyses will uncover any hidden measures that are outside the norm, and needing attention:

> These include a PSA test for cancer of the prostate, cholesterol levels, especially to check for elevated LDL (bad) cholesterol, blood sugar levels to stay ahead of diabetes, liver functions, and the presence of antibodies, which may signal an infection. Depending on the findings, your doctor may refer you to a specialist, like a cardiologist, an endocrinologist for hormonal issues, a urologist for prostate and urinary issues, or a dietician for weight management.
>
> If you're having muscular, skeletal or joint problems, you may need to see an orthopedist. Middle-age men who are experiencing problems with balance and coordination, or back pain, may be directed to a neurologist for evaluation.

Warning: Limit your exams and advice to reputable medical and healthcare professionals. Do not be seduced by the temptations of advertising, offering dramatic weight loss, regaining lost youth, revitalizing your energy, preventing heart disease. Almost none of these products or their claims have been evaluated by the FDA, and are probably not worth the payments you may have been making. Even most vitamin supplements are unnecessary and pass right through you, and are excreted in your urine. We'll cover the subject of micronutrients and supplements in chapter 5.

Okay, we've covered the medical side of things, now we can move on to a more in-depth understanding of how diet and nutrition are influential on health, wellbeing, and your longevity.

Chapter 2: Can Healthy Eating Turn Your Health Around?

In chapter 1, you learned about the health issues that can affect mature men and became familiar with a broad range of potential risks to your health and wellbeing, your quality of life, and your longevity. We also highlighted the lifestyle changes that can make the difference in protecting you from encroaching illnesses and conditions that can disrupt your life, debilitate you, or even threaten your life. Effectively managing your health through the right lifestyle choices can, as we said, put more life into years, and potentially, *add more years to your life*.

Themes and Principles

We can't control everything that affects us, like who our parents were, and the genetic profile we inherited, but we can greatly improve the odds on our behalf.

The recurrent theme is that you can have control over your health and the conditions, diseases and disorders that can threaten it, now that you're a half-century man. You have the ability to turn your health around, become stronger, more resistant to diseases, and able to regain at least some of the energy, vitality, and self-esteem of your earlier years. Instead of surrendering to age, you can take the initiative and manage your coming years proactively and positively.

The underlying principle of ensuring your health and longevity is that among the many lifestyle changes you'll be considering, nutrition and diet—healthy eating—is the singular most important and influential.

So, now we are going to take a deeper dive into nutrition and understand why it is the one lifestyle change that outweighs all the others. You'll learn what you need to know about counting calories (and why you need to place more emphasis on food quality than quantity).

The Respected Resources

To provide the most thorough and up-to-date information on healthy dietary practices for middle-aged men, we have turned to trusted authorities for research-based and experience-based reports and recommendations. These sources have key findings in common, and some divergences. For example, all of the sources emphasize plant-based diets, avoidance of processed foods, and of chemically loaded preservatives. Unprocessed foods, whole grains, vegetables and fruit in abundance, and the reduction or elimination of sugar, and saturated fats; all are common to our sources.

But there are **divergences** when it comes to one subject: meat, fish, and dairy, as animal-sources of protein. Some authorities advocate diets that embrace the *complete elimination of all animal sources* in the diet, and have research and testimonials attesting to disease prevention, disease and illness cures, weight management and greater overall health and wellbeing.

Yet other authorities are less extreme in their requirements. The same plant-based emphasis is present, but there is more tolerance for small quantities of lean meat, fish, and dairy products. As you will see below (Harvard School of Public

Health), meat and fish are appreciably higher in protein than plant-based sources. This makes a vegetarian diet (no meat, poultry or fish, but dairy and eggs are okay) or vegan diet (pure plant foods vegetarian, no exceptions for dairy and eggs) more challenging to achieve adequate protein.

What to do? Become knowledgeable, and make informed decisions based on your own preferences. The recurring concept of the quality of the foods you eat is consistent throughout all of the studies and recommendations.

The 80:20 Principle

There's a popular expression among nutritionists, "You can't outrun your fork," cited by Terri Edwards in *T. Colin Campbell Center of Nutrition Studies* (2018). It means, quite literally, is that diet is four times as influential than exercise in weight loss. This is not to diminish or disparage exercise, but the intent is to quantify the effects of diet as the prevailing influence. This is no idle cliché, but is based on solid research.

There are several science-based reasons that most weight loss comes from diet. First, science is overwhelmingly in agreement that weight gain, weight maintenance, and weight loss, are entirely a function of **calories in, and calories out**. It's as much physics as it is biology. The first law of thermodynamics states that matter can neither be created nor destroyed.

Applying this concept to weight control, if you consume 3,000 calories in one day, and burn (through metabolism) 2,000 calories that same day, you will have a net gain of 1,000 calories. It doesn't matter how you burned those calories, and if you continue the same pattern, in four days you will have accumulated 4,000 extra calories, enough to add one pound of weight (it takes about 3,500 calories per pound gained).

Next, **it takes a lot of exercise** to burn a relatively small amount of calories, thanks to our having evolved a very efficient energy-conserving body. If you walk an extra five miles in a day, you will burn 500 calories, and have, for the moment, a 500 calorie deficit. but as soon as you pop some food in your mouth, that 500 calorie deficit is done. One cheeseburger will do it easily. Even a simple grilled cheese sandwich, with 200 calories in two slices of bread, and another 300 calories in three small square slices of American or Swiss cheese. Ice cream? A ¾ cup serving of one of the more expensive brands (which are denser and higher in fat) will easily add about 350 calories to your daily total.

Dietician and fitness authority Albert Matheny, Rd, CSCS, sums it up nicely, saying that weight loss depends on maintaining a *negative energy balance*. We can interpret this concept with the simple example of a bag of marbles. The weight of the bag varies entirely on how many marbles are added, and how many are taken away. It doesn't matter what color or design, as long as each marble weighs the same as the others.

Calories are like that. One gram of carbohydrates or protein contains four calories, regardless of the source; one gram of fat or oil contains nine calories (nature's way of efficiently conserving energy).

Assistant professor Holly Lofton, who directs the weight management program at NYU's Langone Medical Center, calculates that you would have to run or walk between seven and 10 miles every day for a week to lose just one pound, and that assumes no increase in calories. Very few people could handle that much exercise, especially men whose knees and joints would be seriously challenged.

Yet another, and rather surprising finding is that primates (humans, apes) tend to maintain the same daily net metabolic rate, regardless of exercises. Studies were conducted among bush people, who are hunters and gatherers still active in remote parts of southern Africa. The researchers compared the daily caloric burn of the bush people to the energy expenditures of sedentary people in America. Despite the differences in daily activity, there was little difference in calories burned per day. Moreover, regardless of variations in daily activities, a person's net caloric burned remained the same each day:

> A leading interpretation of these findings is that the body adjusts to keep the daily metabolic rate consistent, regardless of how little or much exercise takes place.

> This suggests that when we exercise a lot on a given day, our metabolism slows down at other times, even when we're sleeping, to compensate.

> The net conclusion is that reducing caloric consumption can be a simple, straightforward way to lose weight. However, everything is not so simple when not all calories are equal to calories. For example, the 140 calories from a 12 oz can of Coca Cola is not a better option compared to 250 calories from the whole avocado. Although the soda beverage will provide you with fewer calories, it will not help you to

lose weight or improve your health. This is directly related to the nutritional quality of the foods consumed being more important than quantity.

Support the concept of quality over quantity, a widely-regarded documentary film, "Forks Over Knives" (2011), revealed a completely new perspective on disease prevention through changes in nutritional practices, notably the elimination of processed foods, and meats, and other animal-derived foods, and their replacement with plant-sourced foods, and unprocessed, whole foods. The concept evolved from the research of two eminent scientists:

- Dr. T. Colin Campbell, Cornell University biochemist
- Dr. Caldwell Esselstyn, Cleveland Clinic surgeon

While their work was conducted independently, their findings converged with the same conclusions: that major diseases can be prevented, or even reversed with natural, whole, grains and other plant-derived foods. The chronic diseases they believed could be prevented include arthritis, type 2 diabetes, heart disease, and cancer. Admittedly, that's quite a claim, so let's look at the research that it's based on.

Results of a study among arthritis patients were published in the medical journal, *Arthritis,* in 2015. It was a randomized, controlled study among osteoarthritis sufferers. One sample continued their normal meat-based diet, the other matched sample ate a meat-free, plant-based diet. After two weeks, the plant foods-only diet followers had a significant reduction in pain, and reported increased functionality. The meat-eating control group did not experience any improvements.

The *Journal of Nutrition, Health and Aging* published an earlier study in 2006 (before the documentary was released), in which people were divided into groups that either, (1) ate meat once a week, or (2) ate meat multiple times per week, or (3) ate no meat, and consumed plant-based foods exclusively. Among men, the meat once-a-week group had a 19% chance of developing osteoarthritis compared to the no-meat, plants-only group. Those who ate meat several times per week had a 43% greater likelihood of developing osteoarthritis.

Based on these and other studies of plant-based, high fiber, meat-free diets, the researchers believe the results are due, at least in part, to reduced weight, which resulted in preventing obesity, and a calming of the immune system, leading to a lowering of chronic inflammation.

Additional evidence is provided, based on individual testimonials, by people who were inspired by the *Forks Over Knives* film, and who came to increased recognition of ethical concerns about eating animals, health concerns about red meat, and a sensitivity to the meat production industry's impact on the environment. This motivated them to try the meat-free, plant-based diet, and they reported weight loss, elimination or reduction of type 2 diabetes, and lower cholesterol levels, leading to lower risk of heart disease, as well as other diseases and conditions.

These findings strongly support the concept that the quality of foods consumed is more important than quantity.

However, endorsers of "Forks Over Knives" principles do not appear to have the backing of large scale, randomized clinical trials to confirm dietary effects in curing or preventing diabetes, heart disease, cancer, and other diseases, as was done for osteoarthritis. In research protocols, individual testimonials are considered *qualitative*, meaning the findings regarding heart disease, diabetes, asthma and other diseases are of directional value, but only a large-scale *quantitative* randomized clinical trial can be considered reliable, and predictive of the likelihood that the results can be repeated. In other words, the testimonials are suggestive, and not statistically significant.

In "A Medical Review of the Documentary Forks Over Knives" (2017), David Hirsch notes that, "While *light on data* from rigorous clinical trials," the film provides ample amounts of what he calls "observational evidence" that many diseases and conditions, including cancer, heart disease, obesity, and diabetes are largely the consequence of a meat-intensive Western diet, and that a plant-based diet can prevent or slow their onset.

The China Study

But Hirsch goes on to cite other studies, including the "China Study," conducted by Drs. T. Colin Campbell and Chen Junshi, which correlated variations in cancer rates in regions of China by the amounts of meat in the diet. According to the researchers, the more meat consumed, the higher the incidences of cancer.

This appears to be a compelling reason to eliminate meat from the diet. Yet the American Institute for Cancer Research (AICR), does not go as far as to recommend complete elimination of meat from the diet, and, while recommending diets that are plant-based, with a variety of vegetables, fruits, nuts, whole grains, and plant oils (especially olive oil), the AICR says it's okay to include fish, limited amounts of red meat and dairy, and poultry:

> The AICR recommends that each meal should be composed of two/thirds plant-based foods, and one-third (or less) of animal-derived foods.
>
> Separate studies strongly advocate the inclusion of cold-water fish in diets for men like us, who are over 50, and most others as well. Fish is valued for low saturated, beneficial fats that are rich in omega-3 antioxidants, and is recommended as a high protein replacement for meat.

To sum up the evidence so far, a diet that is largely (if not exclusively) based on plant-derived foods (vegetables and salads, whole grains, nuts and seeds, oils, unprocessed cereals), and is low in dairy, meats, and other animal-sourced foods, can play a major role in disease prevention, weight control, and overall health and wellbeing. What is frequently ignored by men in America is the overall quantity and quality of the foods we consume. There is some truth to the expression, "You are what you eat."

Benefits of a Healthy Diet

The *Men's Health Forum* is a valuable resource for easy to understand ways to improve your health through diet and nutrition. You'll find a link to their website in the References section, for easy access. It's a well-organized, informative site. The benefits of a healthy diet are both short-term and long-term, and are interpreted here. Let's start with the more immediate, short-term benefits:

Appearance. This includes activity and appearance benefits like getting you into good shape overall, and keeping you there, and improving how your external features are optimized, including your eyes and vision, your skin, even the appearance and condition of your nails and hair.

Energy. Eating right gives you energy and endurance on both physical and mental levels, so you can get up and go, and workout and keep up with the younger guys. At the same time, your mind will benefit, with greater concentration, improved memory, and a more positive state of mind.

Immunity. Diet contributes to a more effective immune system, so invading pathogens, like bacteria and viruses, will be met promptly and powerfully with the initial, innate immune response, which detects and destroys these threats. If you do become sick, a strong immune system will speed your recovery.

Digestion. You can avoid constipation, diarrhea, irritable bowel syndrome (IBS) and other digestive malfunctions by eating the foods that keep things moving smoothly through the digestive tract. The right diet nourishes the trillions of beneficial bacteria and other microbes in the gut microbiota.

Longer-Term. Over time, good nutrition can help lower the risk of cardiovascular diseases like atherosclerosis (buildup of plaque in the coronary arteries) and hypertension (high blood pressure), and prevent obesity, which can lead to the onset of type 2 diabetes. By avoiding the saturated fats of meat, especially beef, LDL (bad) cholesterol levels can be lower, and beneficial HDL cholesterol can be elevated.

The right diet can also reduce the risk of certain types of cancer, and head off osteoporosis, by ensuring you are ingesting the most beneficial foods, and avoiding those with potentially injurious ingredients.

Eating the right foods over the long haul will continue to keep you in better shape overall, and help maintain good health. In addition to supporting the immediate, innate immune system, over time a good diet will also improve the important secondary, or **adaptive immune system,** which manages the more challenging viruses and other pathogens that are not stopped initially. The adaptive immune response includes the cytokines interferon and interleukin, which detect viruses, and send signals to trigger the 'killer 'B cells and T cells that prevent viruses from invading cells and replicating, and also lead to the formation of antibodies that protect against future infections of the same virus. In other words, immunity.

Harvard School of Public Health

Another excellent source of valuable guidance and information on diet and nutrition is Harvard University's T.H. Chan School of Public Health, which is the successor to a century of investment in dietary and health research. As public health became a greater priority, the School of Public

Health separated from Harvard Medical School and became an independent educational institution, increasing its ability to proactively engage in all aspects of public health, wellbeing and longevity. With a large staff of professional researchers and scientists, the School is a leading source of new concepts and ideas in nutrition and diet that affect health, quality of life, living longer and better.

Harvard's School of Health has a very informative website, which you can access from the link in the References (Harvard T.H. Chan. 2020). Here is the School of Health's excellent definition of carbohydrates, proteins and fats. We've touched on this before, and will again, but this can stand as definitive:

Carbohydrates are composed of carbon and hydrogen, primarily (as the name implies), and are the body's primary source of energy. Despite the bad press that 'carbs 'have been receiving, in reality, they are an essential part of a healthy diet, by providing glucose, a chemical derivative of sugar that is converted to the energy that the cells need to enable us to perform activities, as well as supporting certain bodily actions and functions. Our bodies create glucose by breaking down sugars, starches, and fibers that we ingest.

Common sources are cereals, breads, and other grain-based foods, as well as cookies and pastries, pasta, and anything made from wheat, rye or other types of flour. We also get carbohydrates from vegetables and potatoes, oatmeal, rice, quinoa, barley, and other cereals, as well as from beans and lentils, which are called legumes.

Within this array, the quality of carbohydrates varies greatly, and some sources are more nutritious and healthier than others; often, the quality of the carbohydrate you consume is more important than the amount, or the percentage of carbohydrates in the daily diet.

To select: Healthy carbohydrates include unprocessed (or minimally processed) whole grains, which have not been stripped of the bran and germ, which are where the essential nutrients, fiber, minerals, vitamins, and even protein are stored. These include whole-wheat breads and pasta, and whole-grain barley, oatmeal, rye, quinoa, and buckwheat. Beans are another good source of carbohydrates and are a good vegetative source of protein.

In addition, vegetables of many types and colors, and fruits are an essential part of a healthy diet, and provide vitamins, minerals and phytonutrients. The different colors of vegetables and fruits are caused by the presence of different nutrients, so a mix of colors is advised.

To avoid. Conversely, carbohydrates to avoid are in refined white flour breads and pasta, and foods like French fries, which are unhealthy for several reasons, including removal of the nutritious outer skin when peeled, and absorption of high-calorie oils and dangerous trans fats during the frying process (the same concerns about frying apply to fried chicken, doughnuts, and all other fried foods).

Importantly, refined carbohydrates, including refined starches and sugars, are absorbed too quickly, and can add to blood sugar spikes, cause weight gain, and lead to the onset of type 2 diabetes.

Harvard School of Public Health recommends a "Healthy Eating Plate," which has vegetables and fruit filling about half the plate, and whole grains, like rice or whole-grain pasta or quinoa, filling another one-quarter of the plate, leaving the remaining quarter for a healthy source of protein (coming up next).

Protein is the building block that our bodies are constructed from muscle, skin, our bones, hair, and virtually every organ and body part. Protein is a key part of enzymes, which mediate chemical reactions, and it forms the hemoglobin in your blood that transports oxygen to the cells. Harvard School of Public Health estimates there are over 10,000 different types of proteins, each carrying out a specific function.

If your body was a car, carbohydrates would be the fuel, and proteins would form primary structural parts of the physical car: the steel, glass, copper, rubber.

Understanding how diet affects protein development requires getting to know about amino acids, which are the building blocks that connect to form the long, complex protein molecules. There are 20 amino acids, and our bodies can combine nutrients to form 14 of them, but nine, called essential amino acids, need to be provided by the food we eat.

You may recognize some of these nine essential amino acids: histidine, methionine and leucine, plus isoleucine, phenylalanine and lysine, threonine, valine, and tryptophan. You won't see them listed on food ingredients, so it's important to know where they can be found in basic, natural sources of protein.

Most meat and fish servings, and egg whites contain all the essential amino acids, but plant-derived foods do not, with rare exceptions (soybeans, notably). Thus, in a classic example, a dish that combines rice (or other cereal) with beans, brings together the nine essential acids to form nutritionally complete protein. We will get into this in more detail in the next chapter.

Protein needs. To ensure we get enough protein every day to meet our building and rebuilding needs, the National Academy of Medicine has determined that seven grams of protein are needed per 20 pounds of weight. So a person weighing 100 pounds needs about 35 grams of protein, a 150-pound person needs about 53 grams, and a 200-pound person needs about 70 grams.

You can see the protein quantity in packaged foods, which show both grams and the percentage of average adult daily requirement (ADR). For example, one cup (eight ounces) of skim milk contains 8 grams of protein (16% of ADR), one large egg contains 6 grams of protein (12% ADR), and one can of solid light tuna (an excellent protein source) contains 26 grams of protein (52% ADR). Each of these is a complete protein source.

Among plant-based sources, a serving (¼ cup dry) of brown rice (unprocessed) provides 4 grams of protein (8% ADR), the same amount of quinoa provides 6 grams, (12%), and a ½ cup serving of garbanzo beans provides 7 grams of protein (14% ADR). One cup of fresh or frozen broccoli provides 2 grams of protein (4% ADR), and the same serving of green peas provides 3 grams of protein (6% ADR).

But there is a wide range of daily protein needs as a percentage of total daily diet, but to the surprise of many men, protein should not be the dominant nutrient. That honor belongs to carbohydrates—yes, 'carbs 'should comprise at least half your daily source of calories; actually, closer to 60%. But with both carbohydrates and protein, the *quality* of these nutrients is much more important than the *quantity*. This was confirmed by a Harvard study that followed 130,000 adults for up to 32 years. The study concluded that longevity did not relate to total protein intake, but *did relate to the source* of the protein.

Now, what about fats? While fats should be the smallest portion of the diet, fats are still a very essential dietary component, but again, it's the source that makes the difference, health-wise. We'll cover this next, but in overview, ideal fats are monounsaturated, like olive oil, or polyunsaturated, including sunflower oil, safflower oil, and corn oil. Fats to limit in your diet are saturated, from fatty cuts of meat, and full-fat dairy, including butter, cheese, and margarine.

Now that you have "digested and assimilated" the studies, you are ready to advance to chapter 3, to consider more precisely what you should do to create your own personalized healthy diet.

Chapter 3: What Should I Eat

We've come to the part of the book that is moving from the factual to the practical, from knowledge to choices. By now, you understand the basic food groups, and what their role is in building, maintaining, and energizing our bodies. You recognize that a diet loaded with fatty meats and greasy fried foods is not what you want to be eating, at any age, but most certainly not when you are a middle-age man You know that a diet that is plant-based tends to be healthier than a diet that is loaded with meat and dairy.

Become familiar with the various food groups, and see where dietary necessity coincides with your preferences. But in overview, is there one diet among the many that is accessible, easy to follow, safe and healthy, and broadly recommended by nutritionists, doctors and dietitians? That honor goes to the Mediterranean diet, which will come up from time to time, and will be fully presented in later chapters. For now, let's tackle the key food groups.

Dietary Recommendations By Food Group

Let's continue the carbohydrates, protein, and fats discussion, by going deeper into what specific foods a mature man should be eating to optimize health. The facts of what these food groups are, and what they are for in our bodies are one thing, but putting it all together into what to eat will give you a practical set of options to choose from. There are foods you should eat, and foods you should not eat, but the objective is not to **restrict your choices** as much as it is to **broaden your choices,** based on taste and texture preferences.

Some clarification is in order, since there is going to be some overlap between food groups. No food providing carbohydrates or protein does so exclusively; almost all foods contain carbs, proteins and fats in varying percentages. So you can count on getting a rage of essential nutrients from most foods. However, there are some sources of fats that do not contain any (or barely traces) of proteins or carbohydrates. Notably, oils.

You will read more about this below, in a discussion of the "protein package."

Cholesterol, gluten. Before we begin the food groups, let's get these two popular concerns out of the way.

The presence of cholesterol in food is generally a concern because of the role of LDL (bad) cholesterol in causing heart disease. But according to the Framingham Study, ingestion of cholesterol in foods has not been proven to raise LDL cholesterol levels in the blood. The reason nutritionists and doctors are wary about cholesterol in foods is that it is almost always found in foods that are high in undesirable saturated fats, as in beef, other meats and poultry, and full-fat dairy products. **One egg** has over 60% of a man's daily recommended allowance of cholesterol, but after being 'blacklisted 'for many years, eggs are again recommended (in moderation) as a good source of nutritionally complete protein (six grams). One egg is only 70 calories, and is low in saturated fats, and high in overall nutrition.

Did you know? No plant-derived food contains cholesterol. It only forms in animals, and is found in animal-sourced foods: beef, lamb, pork, poultry, and fish, and dairy and eggs.

What about gluten? This complex protein is formed by two simpler proteins in wheat, rye, spelt and other grains, when dough is kneaded. Gluten is valued by bakers because it provides structure to bread, enabling it to trap expanding carbon dioxide gas as yeast consumes sugars in the dough mixture. Only about 2% of the U.S. population has celiac disease, which is the sensitivity to gluten. This suggests that the current trend of gluten-free foods is an overreaction.

Recommended Carbohydrates

Harvard University's School of Public Health authorities recommend the following ways to eat carbohydrates (plus some good protein) that are beneficial, starting with breakfast, which is an ideal time to get going with wholesome whole grains.

Cereal. Start the day with whole-grain cereals, for the benefits of healthy carbohydrates, plus a good start on the day's protein and fiber intake.

You may be aware that oatmeal has been making a resurgence, especially among men our age, and older, driven by studies that credit oatmeal with lowering LDL (bad) cholesterol. Upon returning to oatmeal now, which we all remember from childhood, mature adults are discovering it tastes good, is easily enhanced with fruits, nuts, yogurt, and other add-ins. It's filling, but without weighing you down.

One serving of oatmeal (½ cup dry) contains 29 grams of sugar-free, healthy carbohydrates, 6 grams of protein, 4 grams of fiber, and is gluten-free. You can double the protein by using low fat or skim milk instead of water. You can raise the protein level even higher with yogurt added in—preferably one of the newly available unsweetened Greek or Icelandic-style yogurts, which are higher in protein than regular yogurt, since much of the water has been filtered out, making these yogurts denser.

Try traditional, 'old-fashioned 'oatmeal, which cooks in just three minutes, and avoid pre-cooked instant oatmeal, which may have lost some nutrients. You can also consider steel cut oats, which have more texture, but just be aware that steel cut oats take about 20-25 minutes to cook. Here are alternatives to cooking:

A new, popular option is to prepare the oatmeal the night before, mixing all the ingredients—oatmeal or steel-cut oats, milk, fresh or dried fruit, nuts, flax seeds, for example—and refrigerating the mix overnight. In the morning, it's ready to eat without cooking, but if you prefer your oatmeal hot, a minute or so in the microwave should warm things up.

If an "out of the box" cold cereal is your preference, avoid the cereals made from refined grains and are loaded with sugar. Read the ingredient list, and look for whole grains as the first ingredient, and also low levels of sugar (less than eight grams in a serving). Traditional corn flakes or whole wheat flakes are good options, as long as they're not sugar-coated.

Bread. It's time for a new perspective on bread. Flour mills began scraping the nutrients of wheat flour kernels before milling, about a century ago, to lengthen storage time. As a result, most of today's bread, rolls, bagels are white bread, made from refined white flour. So as we've been saying, the key nutrients and fiber have been stripped out, leaving the starchy endosperm; essentially, an 'empty' carbohydrate that causes a spike in blood sugar. But breads made with whole grain are nutritious, slow to introduce natural sugar, in the form of glycogen, into the bloodstream.

Be careful; read the list of ingredients, and don't be fooled by claims of 'multigrain, 'which is really a mix of refined flours. A good, readily available option is 100% whole wheat bread.

If you have access to a traditional or artisanal bakery, ask for whole grain breads, especially with added seeds (like flax seeds, sunflower seeds, or millet). If you like rye bread, be aware that most commercially available rye breads list refined white wheat flour as the first ingredient.

For optimal nutrition and taste, try baking your own bread. It's not that difficult, and gives you the opportunity to select every ingredient, keeping things whole, natural, and low in sodium too. Home baked bread tastes great, and you'll feel proud of your accomplishment.

Whole grains. These unground whole grains should play a role in salads, and as part of lunch or dinner menus. There are many versions of rice available today, so you can bypass white rice, which is another grain stripped of its nutrients. Look for brown rice, or some of the newer mixes of brown, red, black and wild rices. As with cereals, choose rice in its natural form, not precooked, for optimal nutrition. Rice cooks in about 20 minutes.

A new, popular alternative whole grain is quinoa, which originated in South America, where it's a staple. Like rice, it comes in various colors, and cooks in about 20 minutes.

One serving of whole grain rice (¼ cup dry) contains 35 grams of sugar-free, healthy carbohydrates, 3 grams of fiber, and 4 grams of protein; quinoa is similar, but with 6 grams of protein. Both grains are gluten-free.

Whole fruit. You may be surprised to learn that eating an orange (or a half grapefruit, or a section of pineapple or melon) is far better for you than drinking the juice. The fruit of the orange provides twice as much fiber as the juice, and less sugar, especially if the juice has added sugar. You have a wide selection of fresh fruit available year round; try to vary the colors of vegetables, which varies the minerals you'll be ingesting.

Vegetables. Most vegetables are primarily carbohydrates, including fiber, and water. Carbohydrates are relatively low in total count, compared to grains, cereals, and fruit. Proteins are present in small amounts, about two to three grams in a serving, so vegetables are best for their minerals, vitamins and other micronutrients.

Potatoes (?) Consumed whole, with the peel, potatoes are a robust source of carbohydrates, plus a small amount of protein and fiber. Most of the fiber is in the peel, which is about 50% fiber. But there are concerns that potatoes are high in carbohydrates relative to other nutrients, and those carbohydrates are the kind that the body digests very quickly, creating a spike in insulin and blood sugar, followed by a steep decline in sugar and insulin. Thus potatoes rate high on the glycemic index.

Yet, other sources report that the protein in potatoes is of higher quality (more essential amino acids than grains, for example). One medium russet potato has four grams of fiber, just over four grams of protein, and virtually no fat. Potatoes are a good source of vitamin C, vitamin B6, and potassium.

In summary, potatoes can be a healthy part of your diet, but in moderation, given the potential high blood sugar concerns.

Beans. These members of the legume family are considered preferable to potatoes, and include beans of every color: black, red, pinto, white, lima beans, and lentils. Beans condense a good amount of nutrition into their compact forms; one cup of combined beans with rice provides 58 grams of carbohydrates, 11 grams of fat, and eight grams of fiber. Beans are also an excellent source of protein, as we'll discuss shortly.

Recommended Plant-Based Proteins

Before covering specific proteins and their qualities in your diet, let's consider the concept of the **protein package,** as defined by Harvard's School of Public Health:

Their studies show that the 'package,' that is, everything that comes with the protein, has more influence than the amount of protein you eat. So, eating healthy proteins from nuts, fish, lean poultry, and legumes like beans, is better in preventing heart disease and other serious diseases, compared to ingesting meats rich in saturated fats, and processed meats, like cold cuts and canned meats.

Okay, let's look at the different plant-based food groups that provide protein.

Vegetables. As explained above, vegetables that go into your salad and onto your dinner plate are low in calories because they are low in all three of the food groups. Those with above average protein include asparagus, artichoke, corn, broccoli, and Brussels sprouts, with about three to four grams of protein per serving.

Whole grains. Just as whole grains are recommended for their quality carbohydrates, they also supply a moderate amount of quality protein. In addition to the familiar oats, wheat, rice and quinoa, there is millet (which is a staple grain in parts of Africa), wild rice, buckwheat (which is not in the wheat family), and lesser known kamut, khorasan, and teff. These grains are of ancient origin and are available in specialty and health foods stores, and national chains like Whole Foods.

Nuts and seeds. You may think of these, especially nuts, as snack foods, and they are healthy snack choices, but consider them too as essential sources of quality protein, fiber, and beneficial antioxidants. Just be aware that nuts and seeds are high in oil, which can raise your calorie count quite easily. Nuts include cashews, pistachios, almonds, pecans, walnuts, macadamia nuts (peanuts are technically a legume).

For example, ¼ cup of walnuts contains four grams of protein and two grams of fiber, plus monounsaturated and polyunsaturated oils. And ¼ cup of pistachios (in shell) contains six grams of protein and three grams of fiber.

Seeds include pumpkin seeds, sunflower seeds, sesame seeds, and, even higher on the nutrient scale, are flax seeds and chia seeds. Two tablespoons of roasted flax seeds contain four grams each of protein and fiber, plus beneficial monounsaturated and polyunsaturated oils, and are rich in antioxidant omega-3 fatty acids.

Legumes. These include some of the "heavy hitters" in the world of plant-based proteins, and include kidney beans, black beans, pinto beans, garbanzo (also known as chickpeas), fava, lentils, and soybeans, which are popularly sold as edamame; they're available fresh and frozen, and also converted to tofu and tempeh. Lower down on the protein scale are green peas, snow peas, split peas. Also, as noted, peanuts belong to the legume family, and are high in protein.

For comparison, while ½ cup of green peas contains two grams of protein and three grams of fiber, ½ cup of beans (pinto, black, white, kidney) is packed with eight grams each of protein and fiber. Peanuts pack eight grams of protein and three grams of fiber into a one ounce serving (about 25 pieces).

Suggestion: Beans and rice, as noted, are an excellent source of carbohydrates and fiber, as well as a very good source of nutritionally complete protein. One cup of beans and rice provides at least 14 grams of protein (which is complete, with all nine essential amino acids). Cooking beans from scratch takes time; ideally, an hour or two of simmering after overnight soaking. Therefore most recipes call for canned beans. These can be a good alternative, but check the label, since most canned beans are high in sodium, which can contribute to water retention, and high blood pressure.

Recommended Meat Proteins

Meat and fish. Okay, welcome to the *heavy-hitter* side of the protein sources. Meat and fish contain much higher amounts of protein, ounce for ounce, than any plant-based sources. Meat includes beef, lamb, pork, and poultry, and fish includes fresh fish of every variety (there are hundreds), as well as canned tuna, sardines, kippered herring, clams and oysters. As reported by Erin Coleman in *Livestrong* (2020), meat (including poultry and fish) contains all 20 of the amino acids (including the nine essential amino acids we cannot produce ourselves) that our bodies need every day to build protein. Meat is classified as a high quality, nutritionally complete protein.

How much protein? As reported by the Academy of Nutrition and Dietetics, for one small, three ounce serving of these popular cuts of meat, including poultry and fish:

- Beef steak, bottom round, protein = 29 grams
- Chicken breast, grilled, protein = 26 grams
- Ground beef, 95% lean, protein = 25 grams
- Turkey, white meat, protein = 25 grams
- Lamb loin, lean cut, protein = 24 grams
- Pork loin, lean cut, protein = 23 grams

- Salmon, sockeye, fresh, protein = 22 grams
- Tuna, yellowfin, canned, protein = 20 grams
- Sardines, canned, protein = 18 grams

Now come the caveats: The protein in meats, poultry and fish, as well as in dairy, is of high nutritional quality, but it's the **protein package** that they are part of that can be troublesome. There are no serious issues with fish, since their fats are healthy, loaded with omega-3 fatty acids. But meat, poultry and animal-sourced dairy products are also accompanied by saturated fats, which, as you now know, can contribute to elevated LDL (bad) cholesterol, leading to atherosclerosis, a buildup of plaque that can clog your arteries.

Meat Protein Cautions

Quality vs. quantity. The Harvard School of Public Health, the American Heart Association, and numerous other authorities advise that meat and poultry in the diet can be excellent sources of protein, but should be consumed in small amounts (three or four ounces, about the size of a deck of cards), no more than twice a week, and in cuts or parts that are lean, and not fatty. Paradoxically, it's the fattier cuts of beef that are the most expensive, because the fat content makes the meat more tender, and to a degree, more flavorful.

Given that the fats in fish are beneficial, these sources of quality protein may be consumed with greater frequency than meats.

But, here too, there are limits. Many types of fish accumulate heavy metals in the ocean, notably mercury, so it's probably best to limit fish to three times per week.

Meats to avoid. You already know about the risks of **saturated fats,** but it's worth repeating that few things you can eat are potentially more injurious to your health. Starting in 1948, and every year since, the many thousands of people being followed by the Framingham Study show evidence that a diet rich in fatty meats can lead to heart disease, eventually resulting in heart attacks, the need for angiograms and insertion of stents to open **clogged coronary arteries**, or, in extreme cases, **open-heart surgery** to replace clogged arteries with arteries transplanted from the legs. If this sounds awful (it is), avoid saturated fats and reduce the risk.

Processed meats. When meat is not trimmed of its saturated fats, and goes from its pure, natural state, and is mixed with chemicals (nitrates, nitrites) for preservation and color, plus salt, sugar, and who knows what, the resultant product is possibly no longer safe to eat.

If you are serious about changing your lifestyle for the better, giving up processed meats altogether is strongly recommended by Harvard, by followers of the Framingham Study, and just about every other health authority. If total absolution is asking too much, then at least resolve to cut back appreciably on these processed, and mostly fatty meats, and if available, choose versions that claim to be minimally processed:

> Frankfurters and hot dogs, bacon, sausages (all kinds: breakfast links, beef, chicken, pork, Italian-style). Also preserved or fermented deli meats that have been chopped, mixed with salt and other ingredients, then reconstituted.
>
> Natural, unprocessed foods are what we evolved to eat.

Recommended Fats and Oils

Here comes the third leg, so to speak, of the nutritional triangle. Oils and fats are the least understood of the three, the most concerning, and yet of great importance to a healthy diet. Just as the protein package can affect the good or bad of certain protein sources, the sources and characteristics of fats and oils vary appreciably in positive and negative values.

Our bodies need fats. According to the American Heart Association (2020), fats give our bodies energy, and provide free fatty acids that are essential in supporting cell growth. Fats protect our organs, keep us warm, and help us absorb fat-soluble vitamins A, D, and E.

As mentioned previously, fat is a compact storage unit for reserved energy. Proteins and carbohydrates contain 4 calories per gram, while fat contains 9 per gram. Evolution selected the fat molecules for their ability to store energy as fat, to be available during times of famine, while not overloading our bodies with excess weight. Of course, today, with two-thirds of the population being overweight or obese, quite a bit of reserved fat is being stored.

Not long ago, food producers shifted to low-fat foods. Even bran muffins reduced their fat content, but there was a cost, because sugar was substituted for the potentially beneficial fats. Refined sugar drives up blood sugar and insulin in a fast spike, followed by a sharp decline. Far better is to select foods with good fats, and avoid the bad fats and oils.

(Let's keep it simple: Fats are oils that are solid at room temperature; oils are the same food, but are liquid at room temperature.)

Quality vs. quantity. Both the Nurses Health Study and the subsequent Health Professional Follow-Up Study prove that there is no connection between the percentage of fat calories, and health, overall. There is no connection between fat *caloric* consumption and heart disease, cancer, and even weight gain. No connection, that is, depending on the *type of fat,* not on the amount of fat.

Good fats. Many decades of studies have established that vegetable oils that are pressed from olives, canola, sunflower seeds, safflower, and corn, as well as from nuts and seeds, are monounsaturated or polyunsaturated, meaning they are easily digested, and appear to prevent the buildup of arterial plaque.

Olive oil, a monounsaturated fat, has emerged in recent years as an ideal fat, and is part of the Mediterranean Diet (which we'll cover in detail).

Bad fats. You know by now that saturated fats are bad for health and longevity. These are the solid, yellowish fats in, and on, beef, parts of poultry, lamb, and pork, as well as in butter, cheese, and ice cream. Notice how these fats are solid at room temperature. These fats are best to avoid, or at least, consume infrequently.

Where possible, remove visible saturated fats before cooking. When it's a well-marbled cut of beef, removal won't be possible–best to avoid fatty meats like this altogether.

When selecting ground beef for hamburgers, meatloaf and meatballs, choose at least 85% lean, or preferably 90% or higher. It may taste a little drier than fatty beef, but your heart will thank you.

Some plant-derived fats are saturated—coconut and palm oils—and may be in some recipes. Use in moderation.

Very bad fats. *Worse than saturated?* Yes, if we're talking about trans fats, which are normally liquid oils that are ultra-saturated by hydrogen to make the oils solid. This is how shortening and margarine traditionally have been made. They are considered a risk for disease and are now being eliminated or replaced. Check the labels of foods and make sure trans fats do not appear in the ingredients list.

Let's wrap up this chapter with a hint of what is to come when we consider and compare various diet options that you have. We've already mentioned the Mediterranean Diet, and you'll be learning why it has emerged as the singular best bet. But first, let's talk about beverages.

Chapter 4: What Should I Drink

Do beverages constitute an important part of a healthy diet, especially if you are a mature man? Yes, of course. For nutrition, and especially for hydration, since we're mostly made of water and need to keep it replenished. But what about all the options available?

Okay, you're thinking, you're not a kid anymore, soft drinks are not a part of your life. You don't think there's sugar, or not much sugar in what you are drinking. Then there's alcohol, and despite all the warnings, haven't you read that alcohol is good for you, something about an ingredient in red wine? Coffee is okay, at least this week, since the good and bad about coffee keeps changing. Tea is supposed to be good for you, but which types?

The point is, it's hard to know what to believe, with conflicting reports and news bulletins, new research replacing older research. Dehydration? We seem to be getting warnings about not getting enough water. Do we need eight glasses a day, 13 glasses a day? Can't we trust our thirst? What about types of water? Mineral water, alkaline water? Bottled water?

Yes, there have been changes, based on research, in what's considered good to drink, and what's not. But not every endorsement of beverages is based on valid research. So this chapter is going to stick with the most trusted sources of solid scientific and medical studies, tests and their findings. We'll start with the subject of sugar, then get into what are nutritious drinks, types of waters, and take on the debatable coffee, and alcohol in all its forms.

Water We Need

"Stay hydrated." This is a common recommendation, and is based on our need to replenish the water that our bodies are made from, and that we continuously expel through sweat, to cool us, and by elimination through urine and bowel movements, to dispose of metabolic waste.

But how much water do we really need? The Mayo Clinic staff (2020) says that water accounts for about 60% of our body weight, and every organ, tissue and cell is dependent on water to function. We can't live without water. In addition to getting rid of wastes, and keeping our temperature within the normal range, water cushions and lubricates our joints, and protects tissues. It forms the plasma in our blood, and the liquid in our lymphatic system.

To avoid the risks of too little water, or dehydration, which is of particular concern for middle-age men, especially when active, the Mayo Clinic recommends a total fluid intake of 13.5 cups, with one cup being eight ounces (240 ml). If that seems like a lot, it is, and we are advised that some of that water requirement is met by drinking coffee, tea, and other beverages, plus is in the foods we eat, especially fruits and vegetables, which are very high in water content.

So, back to the question of how much water do you really need to drink? The Mayo Clinic advises that **eight glasses** (cups) of water, which is a popular recommendation, like an adage, and it turns out to be a pretty good guideline. But the amount you need can vary, depending on the weather, and exercise (both of which can cause excessive sweating, and metabolic activity).

A signal of dehydration. Do not rely on your thirst mechanism to determine when it's time to drink; do it regularly, and keep alert for *dark urine*, which is a *clear sign* that you need more water.

If you prefer bottled water, especially from springs and wells, this will ensure clean, fresh tasting, and non-chlorinated water. Is tap water okay? Yes, virtually everywhere in the U.S., but it may have a chlorinated odor, and usually is fluorinated. A simple water filter can generally purify the water.

Some people advocate alkaline water, since our blood and most of our bodily functions are slightly alkaline, but there is no evidence that consuming alkaline fluids or foods affects the alkalinity of our blood or body. Also, anything we drink (or eat) heads directly to the stomach to begin digestion in a very acidic environment.

A touch of lemon. The Department of Agriculture (USDA) recommends water as the ideal beverage for natural hydration, and suggests a squeeze of lemon in each glass to add some flavor, but without adding sugar or other "empty calories." As a bonus, a small amount of vitamin C will be there for you too.

Sugar in Beverages
More Than You Realize

Let's get started with soft drinks, not just because they are notoriously loaded with refined white sugar, but also so they can provide a frame of reference for other, less obvious beverages where sugar is 'hidden. '

One 12 oz (355 ml) can of **Coca-Cola** contains 35 grams of sugar, which totals 140 calories. More graphically, that's 10 teaspoons of sugar. So two cans of Coke per day for one 30-day month adds up to 2,100 grams of sugar, or, 8,400 calories. Since 3,600 incremental calories add one pound of body weight, that's a potential monthly weight gain of two and one-third pounds. Keep up the incremental Coca-Cola calories for one year, and the weight gain could be 28 pounds.

Impressive? This is one of the reasons two-thirds of American adults are overweight or obese. Just two cans of Coke per day. But soft drinks are certainly not the only beverage with hidden, empty calories from sugar.

Energy drinks pack quite a caloric punch. One small eight oz (240 ml) can of Rockstar Energy Drink has 31 grams of sugar, which contribute 124 calories. Close behind, competitor Red Bull Energy Drink has 27 grams of sugar, and 108 calories.

How about ice tea? Surely this should be less fattening than soda and energy drinks, right? Wrong. Ice tea you make at home can be sugar-free, or lightly sugared, but if you try Arizona Lemon Ice Tea, even an eight oz (240 ml) serving contains 24 grams of sugar, and 100 calories. Prefer Snapple? You'll consume 23 grams of sugar and acquire 92 calories in an eight oz (240 ml) serving.

Vitamin-enriched water should be less sugary, and it is, but is still sneaking in more calories from sugar than you might think. All flavors of Vitamin Water brand contain 52 calories in one eight ounce serving, coming from 13 grams of sugar.

Lemonade? Minute Maid doesn't want the lemons in their lemonade brand to be too bitter, so 27 grams of sugar and their 108 calories are added to an eight oz (240ml) serving.

Okay, at least **fruit juice** is safe, isn't it? Another 27 grams of sugar and 108 calories are found in an eight oz (240 ml) serving of Minute Maid **Orange Juice**. If you can make fresh squeezed orange juice, and add no sugar, your caloric intake will be much lower.

So pay attention to the ingredients on the labels. Look for versions that are unsweetened, or lightly sweetened, with far less sugar and fewer non nutritious calories.

Sports Beverage Surprises. Gatorade was the first to bring what is called isotonic beverages to the public. Today there are many brands, all promising to provide energy, replace electrolytes, and, of course, to hydrate. But medical authorities consider that these specialized beverages are not necessary, except when engaged in extreme sports, with considerable exertion, and heavy sweating.

Sports beverages, like Gatorade and Powerade, contain electrolytes, to replace sodium, potassium, magnesium and calcium, plus minerals, sugar, and amino acids. But are these nutrients necessary for most mature men?

Gatorade contains 50 calories, mostly from sugar, and other brands have up to 150 calories per eight oz (240 ml) serving. This puts them in the category of sugary beverages. Writing in "CNET Health and Wellness" (2020), Amanda Capritto reports that sports drinks are like any other beverage containing sugar, and can contribute to excess calories and, over time, can lead to weight gain. She says that it's generally better to prevent dehydration by drinking water throughout the day and evening, and only using a sports beverage when losing a good quantity of minerals and fluids through heavy exertion and sweating.

The conclusion: You are better off drinking adequate amounts of water when exercising, and during the following recovery period. You probably don't need the extra sugar carbs, and also probably do not need to recharge your electrolytes and amino acids. Be aware of how much you are drinking, and don't trust your thirst to keep you hydrated. If your workout is intensive, you can drink a sports beverage, but don't overdo it, and drink water as well.

Nutritious Beverages

Apple Cider Vinegar

Does apple cider vinegar improve health at any age, especially for men? In popular culture, vinegar is credited with improving heart health, controlling blood sugar levels and helping weight control by burning fat; it has been used in a variety of treatments since ancient times.

Vinegar is produced first by bacterial fermentation of a carbohydrate (like apples) to create alcohol, which is then converted by another type of bacteria to acetic acid. It's the acetic acid that makes vinegar taste bitter and acidic, and which purportedly provides the health benefits.

It's not necessary (or advisable) to drink apple cider vinegar except in small quantities, about one to two tablespoons per day. It's acidic, and you may prefer to have it in salad dressing, or you may drink it diluted in a glass of water.

Here are the benefits attributed to apple cider vinegar. Note that not all benefits have been validated by scientific research protocols:

Heart disease. As reported by Arizona State nutritionists Johnston and Gass in "Medscape General Medicine" (2006), there are suggestive but not conclusive findings that apple cider vinegar prevents heart disease; findings that are mostly obtained from clinical testing with mice. The Nurses' Health Study did record a significantly reduced risk for fatal, ischemic heart attacks among the participants whose diets included oil and vinegar-based salad dressings five or more times per week, but there are no similar findings among adult humans, and specifically for men.

Moreover, there was no way of determining if the results of the Nurses'Health Study are causative or coincidental (in other words, this does not prove that the vinegar was responsible for the benefits). The same source also reported that apple cider vinegar contains polyphenols, which have an antioxidant effect. Other studies testing the antibacterial effects of vinegar did not confirm this benefit.

Antiglycemic effect. There is some clinical data that show reduced blood sugar following a meal high in carbohydrates, and which included salad dressing containing apple cider vinegar. Separately, similar results were achieved with a pickled cucumber, which, like vinegar, is high in acetic acid.

Weight loss. There is limited evidence that apple cider vinegar is directly responsible for weight loss, possibly due to some studies showing that it increases satiety, i.e., feeling of fullness, which can suppress appetite, and lead to lower caloric intake.

Summing up. Mythical beliefs aside, there is no harm in adding apple cider vinegar to your diet, and there are possibilities that yet-unproven health benefits may accrue. But do not rely on vinegar to be a cure-all, able to offset the negative effects of a bad diet, and lack of exercise.

Coffee is Approved

Coffee is surviving the controversies, and is currently considered a beneficial beverage, providing a number of healthful benefits. Most of the negative reports tended to arise from metadata studies, which combine numerous studies to reach overarching conclusions. For example, coffee has been found to be consumed by men who have heart disease, but that is not proof that there is a cause and effect relationship. That a man who has heart disease happens to drink coffee may be purely coincidental.

Here are recent findings that can put coffee drinkers at ease, reported by Nikki Jong in "One Medical" (2017), and which we've summarized:

> **Antioxidant**. Coffee can calm inflammation because of its antioxidant qualities. More than 1,000 antioxidants are found in coffee beans, and even more develop during roasting. Coffee is higher in antioxidants than black tea, green tea, and cacao. Chlorogenic acid is a potent antioxidant that is found only in coffee, and is credited with preventing cardiovascular disease. Overall, antioxidants neutralize free radicals, which are destructive byproducts of the metabolic process in cells. Antioxidants are also credited in preventing chronic (long lasting) disorders, ranging from arthritis to certain types of cancer.
>
> **Cognitive health**. A study in Finland showed that cognitive decline, especially Alzheimer's disease, can be slowed by

drinking coffee. Those who drank from three to five cups of coffee daily during their midlife years, were 65% less likely to develop Alzheimer's disease and other cognitive disorders, later in life. Tea drinkers did not experience the same benefits. A leading theory is that caffeine slows the formation of beta amyloid plaque in the brain, which disrupts neural connections. Another possible explanation is the reduced tendency to develop type 2 diabetes, which is often associated with cognitive decline.

Memory enhancement. An Austrian study found that the caffeine in one cup of coffee (about 100 mg) increased brain activity while subjects were performing memory tasks. Reaction times and memory were improved relative to a control group that consumed a placebo instead of caffeine. Functional MRI (fMRI) brain scans confirmed these findings. The effects on memory may be short term, however, and the effects may vary from person to person.

Heart health. In yet another European study, a large clinical trial involving more than 37,000 subjects, over a 13 year period in the Netherlands, found that drinking two to four cups of coffee per day conferred a 20% lower risk of developing cardiovascular disease, compared to non-drinkers and light drinkers of coffee, as well as compared to heavy coffee drinkers. While not yet fully confirmed, it appears that the arteries are being protected from inflammatory damage.

Prostate cancer prevention. A study conducted by the Harvard School of Public Health found that men who drink coffee have a reduced risk of developing aggressive forms of prostate cancer, and other forms of cancer, including colon, rectal and liver, as well as helping prevent endothelial and breast cancer in women. Credit is given to antioxidant polyphenols in coffee, which prevent inflammation that is conducive to the growth of tumors.

Preventing diabetes. Two studies demonstrate coffee's role in helping slow or stop the adult onset of type 2 diabetes. One study in 2009 showed a seven percent reduction in risk for every one cup of coffee consumed per day. An earlier epidemiological study indicated that men who drank five or more cups of coffee per day had a 50% lower risk of diabetes, compared to light and non-drinkers of coffee. The explanation for these effects is traced to the regulation of insulin production and sugar levels in the blood. An ingredient unique to coffee—caffeic acid—is believed to prevent the buildup of toxic proteins called amyloid fibrils, which may cause diabetes. Interestingly, for this last benefit, decaffeinated coffee confers the same positive results.

Liver health. The Archives of Internal Medicine includes a study that proves that coffee drinking helps prevent cirrhosis of the liver, including cirrhosis caused by alcohol. A reduction of 20% is credited to each cup of coffee per day, to a maximum of four. The coffee is believed to lower the level of toxic liver enzymes, which can cause inflammation.

Enhanced exercise. Coffee is well recognized as a source of energy, due to caffeine's boosting of blood sugar, and this can appreciably reduce fatigue and increase endurance. Some trainers and coaches believe that coffee can lead to dehydration, but recent research refutes this. Coffee also helps muscle contractions and reduces the person's perception of pain. Up to five cups of coffee per day are recommended for improved performance.

Antidepressant. Coffee drinkers have been found through studies to be at least 20% less likely to be depressed, compared to non-drinkers of coffee. Whether this is causative or coincidental is not yet understood, but the caffeine in coffee is known to activate serotonin and dopamine, which are mood-enhancing neurotransmitters.

Autoimmune prevention. Overactivity by our immune systems can lead to chronic inflammation, and that can wreak havoc on our joints, causing rheumatoid arthritis, gout, and other disorders. The caffeine in coffee has been found to prevent inflammation, and as reported in "Arthritis & Rheumatism," men consuming five cups of coffee per day reduced the likelihood of gout by 40%. Coffee's antioxidant properties may reduce insulin production, which can raise uric acid levels, the cause of gout.

What about tea? Both black tea, and green tea, are a recognized source of antioxidants, but as noted above, coffee is higher in antioxidants than either. However, tea has qualities beneficial to health. According to the Harvard School of Public Health assistant professor Qui Sun, tea contains polyphenols, which provide anti-inflammatory and antioxidant benefits. As cited in Harvard Health Publishing (2014), professor Qi advises that tea, like coffee, can be part of an overall healthy diet and lifestyle to help prevent heart disease and other serious disorders. For those who simply do not like coffee and prefer tea, many of the benefits of coffee are possible.

Bottom line. Coffee may be enjoyed by men without concerns for whether it is good or bad for you. Certainly its positive qualities, when combined with the enjoyment and energy boost it provides, far outweigh any negatives.

But as with anything else, don't overdo it; the same caffeine in coffee that gives you an energy boost can give you jitters if you drink too much. Some of us may find coffee acidic, leading to gastric distress, and acid reflux. Find your comfort zone, and don't overdo it.

Don't drink coffee after dinner or towards bedtime, since its energy boost can lead to insomnia, elevated pulse rate, and higher blood pressure. Remember that coffee is a stimulant, and its effects can last up to six hours.

Alcohol: Facts and Fictions

Alcohol in Moderation

We touched on this key recommendation in chapter 1, and it's a good starting point for this more in-depth examination. In recommending moderation, the intent is not to encourage non-drinkers to start drinking, as if you are missing out on some miracle ingredient or beneficial effect. Alcohol has many dangers, and for some people, the risks outweigh any possible pleasures or physical benefits. So if you are middle age and you have not been a drinker of alcoholic beverages, it's best not to start now.

This is confirmed by the Mayo Clinic (2020), which says that any possible benefits of alcohol are "relatively small" and it is not advised for anyone to start drinking alcohol, or increase current levels if the person is already a moderate drinker, in expectation of enhanced health benefits. The potential "benefits do not outweigh the risk."

Light to moderate drinkers can "probably continue" to drink alcohol responsibly, the Mayo Clinic staff concludes.

Okay, that said, if you drink, most authorities recommend that adult men of all ages should limit their consumption to two drinks per day, and at least one resource says that limit should be one drink per day for men over 65.

But the CDC and other authorities caution that we should limit our weekly alcohol consumption, as well as the daily amount. One source recommends no more than 15 drinks per week for men, (which would accommodate the 2-drinks-a-day guideline) and another, more conservative source proposes a "1-2-3 rule," which recommends either one, or at most, two drinks in a day, but in total, drinking should be limited to three times a week. This would put a six-drinks-per-week limit on male drinkers.

One drink is a 5 ounce glass of red or white wine, or a 12 ounce glass of beer, or a 1.5 ounce serving of distilled spirits, like vodka, gin, tequila, rum, bourbon, rye, scotch, or other type of whiskey.

Many studies find that moderate drinking can be beneficial. The Mayo Clinic staff, writing in "Alcohol Use: Weighing the Risks and Benefits" (2020), says that health benefits of moderate consumption may:

> Reduce the risks of heart disease, potentially reducing risks of a blocked artery in the

brain (ischemic stroke), and may even help prevent the onset of type 2 diabetes.

But the staff qualifies those findings, by saying that there is far more evidence that a nutritious, healthy diet and physical exercise will provide greater health benefits than alcohol. Caution seems to be the watchword when considering alcoholic beverages.

You may have heard about an ingredient in red wine, resveratrol, which is an antioxidant, and its health benefits, especially in preventing heart disease. The American Heart Association (2019), reports that a cause and effect connection between drinking red wine, or any form of alcohol, and improved heart health, has not been established, but there is an association between moderate drinking and a lower risk of death from heart disease.

The AHA cites Dr. Robert Kloner, Huntington Medical Research Institutes senior science officer, and director of cardiovascular research. (He is also a professor of medicine at the University of Southern California). Kloner says that it's not clear whether red wine has a direct role in providing benefits, or whether red wine drinkers just happen to follow a Mediterranean diet, which he says "is cardio-protective." All forms of alcohol, not just red wine, seem to confer some cardio-protective benefits, Kloner says. There are no unique benefits to any particular form of beverage; alcohol is the same carbohydrate, with the same effects.

Alcohol: The Downsides

Heavy drinking, which is three or more drinks a day, can be seriously detrimental to health and longevity. Be especially careful not to overdo the drinking, and never allow yourself to get drunk. Avoid 'binge 'drinking, when a night is spent drinking to excess, and five or more drinks are consumed within two hours.

Never drive a vehicle after drinking more than one drink, under any circumstances, and preferably, avoid alcohol altogether before taking the wheel. Have a non-drinker in your group act as designated driver, or call a taxi or Uber (or Lyft) driver to get you home.

It's important to avoid drinking distilled spirits 'straight,' as in tequila shots, for example. Why? Over 50, your esophagus doesn't appreciate the 'burn 'of direct contact with alcohol, and over time, straight, undiluted spirits can lead to gastroesophageal damage, or cancer. Serve "on the rocks," or mixed with water or other beverages. It's safer, and you'll get more of a taste experience.

What about beer? It's the oldest form of fermented beverages, having been consumed (and enjoyed) for well over 10,000 years. It's low in alcohol compared to wine and distilled spirits, and actually contains traces of vitamin B. But rumors are circulating about "beer boobs" (sagging breasts), and "brewer's droop" (impotence); two physical negative side-effects of beer drinking. These effects are said to be caused by the hops in IPA beer, in particular. Not to worry; these claims have been disproved, and can be ignored. While the hops in beer do contain a plant ingredient, a phytoestrogen, the levels are far too low to have any physical effects. This is confirmed by professor of medical chemistry, Richard van Breemen, at the College of Pharmacy of the University of Illinois. He says, "There is a minute quantity of an estrogen-like compound, 8-prenylnaringenin, in hops...but the levels are too low to be a hormone disruptor."

The Mayo Clinic lists these possible health consequences of excessive drinking for men; these are worth thinking about when considering taking that third glass of wine or whiskey:

- Cancer of the oral cavity (mouth, throat), esophagus, and liver.
- Pancreatitis and liver disease, including cirrhosis.
- Cardiovascular disease, including heart muscle damage; a condition called alcoholic myopathy, and which can lead to heart failure, when insufficient blood is pumped by the heart.
- If you already have heart disease, heavy drinking may cause heart attacks and strokes from high blood pressure.
- Injuries caused by impaired judgment, and depression, potentially leading to suicide.

It's worth noting amazing things that happen when you drink less alcohol (Team Legion, 2019):

- You'll probably lose weight, because alcohol contains what's called empty calories; pure carbs with no nutritional value, and which are absorbed and assimilated before the more nutritious complex carbohydrates, proteins and fats. Skip two drinks and save 300 calories or more.
- You'll lower the risk of heart disease. Really? Alcohol does not contain LDL (bad) cholesterol, but too much alcohol can raise

your LDL cholesterol levels. Plus, those empty calories add up fast, and contribute to weight gain.

- You'll sleep better. Despite alcohol's short-term effect of slowing you down and making you drowsy, drinking before sleeping disrupts restorative brainwaves, and messes with Rem sleep, when dreaming occurs. Plus, it's a diuretic, which means more mid-sleep interrupts to hit the toilet.

- You'll enhance your brainpower. Be aware that heavy drinking can induce changes in the brain that diminish your ability to learn how to solve problems and to learn from mistakes. Cutting back, or cutting out, the drinking can restore those key functions.

- You'll gain and rebuild muscle. Your body will do that naturally after your workout, but not if alcohol gets in the way. Studies show that alcohol interferes with the production of protein and new muscle tissue, and diminishes the human growth hormone.

- You'll boost your immune system. Within 20 minutes of ingesting alcohol, the ability of your immune system to react to invading pathogens is diminished, leaving you more susceptible to infection.

Okay, time to move on to the micronutrients, vitamins, minerals, and the various supplements that may enhance our health. Or do they? Let's see.

Chapter 5: Micronutrients and Supplements

Do we need them? Do we need the vitamins and minerals, the hormones, the amino acids, the herbal extracts, and all the other supplements available to us every day in advertising in every form of media, and on the shelves in pharmacies, supermarkets, health food stores, and of course in stores specializing in supplements?

Does a Mature Man Need Supplements?

Yes and no. Or so it seems. We can assume that no diet is perfect, and perhaps something is missing that can be supplied easily with a micronutrient or supplement. Or, we may assume that the diets of many mature men have serious deficiencies, and supplements are important to maintain good health. As you will see, our bodies are changing, our hormones are declining, our needs are evolving. Can we get everything we need from our diets?

Let's take vitamin D. It's essential for strong bones, and we are expected to get our daily ration from milk and dairy products, and from sunlight. But what if you are off dairy products (or limited), and, aren't we supposed to avoid sunlight, to prevent skin cancer? Or what if you live in an area where it's rainy and overcast much of the time? (The Pacific Northwest comes to mind.) It's a dilemma, perhaps easily resolved by taking a small vitamin D capsule every day. But is it necessary for you?

If you follow a vegetarian, or especially a vegan diet, you probably need to supplement your diet with vitamin B-12, since it is not supplied by plant-based foods. But does this apply to you, with your particular diet?

For most of us, micronutrients and supplements are a temptation (advertising entices us), but are they a necessity? As a mature man you have nutritional needs that are not the same as when you were younger. Nutrients may not be absorbed as easily. We don't want to overeat, just to get the nutrients, the vitamins and minerals, that we need. What about testosterone, which we know is not what it used to be? How can you tell if it's time to get the testosterone checked, and supplemented?

As with the other aspects of good nutrition we've been reviewing, there are lots of opinions and information sources to tell us what supplements we need. Let's focus on the recommendations of the competent authorities. Just the facts, please.

Are Supplements Necessary?

The issue is not purely "yes or no" when it comes to supplements; it's more a case of confirming necessity rather than assuming a daily supplement, like a multivitamin, is a requirement for all of us.

Let's begin with a perspective from Donald B. McCormick, Ph.D., who is a professor emeritus of biochemistry at Emory University. He says that while half of adults who are age 65 or above take supplements and vitamins every day, he questions whether most of them are needed. McCormick thinks that for the typical mature man, most essential nutrients can be obtained by adjusting diet. He believes that "A lot of money is wasted," on supplements that are unnecessary. He questions the increased need for vitamins and minerals as we age, saying that there is insufficient research to justify the expenses incurred, and that supplements do not "cure the aging process."

McCormick is at odds with research findings that recommend that older adults need two daily multivitamins. He saw no proof that seniors need more niacin, riboflavin, or thiamin as they mature, but acknowledges some may need more folate, vitamin B6, and B12.

So, it's worth questioning the need for supplements, and being targeted on specific needs, rather than a 'shotgun, 'all-inclusive approach.

Fortified Foods

As an alternative to supplements, your age-induced increased needs for vitamins and minerals may be met through a combination of fresh foods, plus packaged foods that have been fortified. The Academy of Nutrition and Dietetics, in their journal "Eat Right" (2020), states that seniors, both men and women, need to ensure they are getting enough calcium and vitamin D, which they can obtain through low-fat (or no-fat) dairy, fortified cereals and fruit juices, dark leafy vegetables, canned fish and fortified plant-based foods. Vitamin D is available in fatty cold-water fish, like salmon, as well as eggs, and fortified beverages, including milk.

It's important to read the labels on packaged foods. Federal regulations in the U.S. and most other countries require listing the nutrients, including overall calories per serving, amounts in grams of carbohydrates, protein, fats, as well as amounts of fiber, vitamins and minerals. The recommended daily allowances for an average adult are also shown, making it easier to see if you are meeting your requirements. Be sure to check the sodium levels and be careful not to overdo the sodium.

But the "average adult" is not necessarily a mature man who is 40 or older and package label information may not be specific to your needs. More to the point, what's good for a 30-year-old may not be relevant to you. This sets up our discussion of supplements.

Playing It Safe with Supplements

Do men over the age of 40 need supplements to replace what is being lost naturally?

An entire industry has been built around the concept that we may not be getting all we need of vitamins, minerals and other micronutrients from the foods we eat. It is suggested, primarily by the producers and purveyors of supplements, but echoed by a variety of opinion-providers, that we don't get all we need from what we eat.

Why are diets deficient? Dietary practices, for one. Skipped meals, unbalanced meals, too many calories from sugar and refined carbohydrates, and fatty meat, and processed meat with saturated fats, at the expense of whole grains and vegetables, good oils and fish, and other foods that can provide vitamins, minerals and other nutrients.

Does your age make a difference? Men of your age may not absorb vitamins and minerals as well as younger men, yet the need for these micronutrients remains the same.

Let's take a realistic look at what you may be missing, just in case your diet choices and practices may leave you below the recommended amount of key nutrients.

Calcium and vitamin D. If you know that you are not getting either of these, you should consider a calcium supplement, and a vitamin D capsule; typically a 1,000 IU capsule of vitamin D3. Alternatively, you may choose a multivitamin, which includes both.

Vitamin B12. As mentioned, those on meatless and fishless diets will need a vitamin B12 supplement. In addition, those of us above age 50 may be challenged to absorb sufficient vitamin B12. You're on the right track if your daily diet includes fortified cereals, meat or fish (including most forms of seafood), but it's a good idea to check with your physician or a dietician, who can determine if you need to take a vitamin B12 supplement. A multivitamin may include B12 among the many others.

Potassium. This mineral is an electrolyte, but unlike sodium (also an electrolyte), potassium does not raise blood pressure. Adequate quantities may be achieved if your diet includes fresh vegetables and fruit, beans and other legumes, and dairy products, especially low-fat or fat-free milk and yogurt.

Fiber. This complex carbohydrate is essential for good digestion, including keeping the gut microbiota nourished and functioning. Fiber is associated with lowering LDL (bad) cholesterol, and reducing the risk of heart disease, as well as type 2 diabetes. A diet containing whole grain breads and cereals, and fruit and vegetables, may provide adequate fiber, but if you are constipated, there are supplements that can increase the daily fiber. Those that provide supplemental fiber in natural form are called *prebiotics* (not to be confused with *probiotics*, which deliver beneficial bacteria to the gut).

How Much Do You Need?

We checked with the NIH's National Institute on Aging to verify how much is needed when deciding if you may need to supplement your diet with vitamins and minerals:

Vitamin B12. You need 2.4 micrograms daily. The NIH counsels that If you're being treated with medication for acid reflux or GERD, there may be a need for a different form. Your healthcare provider will be able to advise you. When you read the information on a supplement package, make sure the amount of vitamin B12 is not excessive.

Calcium. Men from age 50 to 70 need 1,000 milligrams, and 1,200 milligrams daily after 70, but check the ingredient on supplements to not exceed more than 2,000 milligrams per day. Get an idea from the milk and egg cartons to get an ideal how much calcium you're getting already from food sources: one cup of milk supplies 25% of your daily calcium; one egg provides just 2%.

Vitamin D. NIH recommends 600 International Units (IU) for men aged 51 to 70 and 800 IU for those over 70, not to exceed daily consumption of 4,000 IU. A supplement for vitamin D is probably a safe way to ensure adequate intake, especially since there's no way to know how much you're getting from sunlight, and food sources may fall short: one cup of milk supplies 15% of your daily vitamin D; one egg provides 6%.

Vitamin B6. For all men, the recommended amount is 1.7 mg for men.

Antioxidants. We normally think of foods as the source of antioxidants, which play a key role in stopping free radicals and preventing inflammation and other chronic disorders. These are the common dietary sources:

> **Vitamin C** is water soluble and provided by citrus fruits and berry fruits, tomatoes (which is a fruit) and peppers.
>
> **Vitamin E** is oil soluble and is provided by nuts and seeds, wheat germ, olive oil, canola oil and peanut oil.
>
> **Beta-carotene** is proved by fruits and vegetables, especially dark green, like spinach, kale, broccoli, and those that are orange, notably carrots.

According to NIH, based on current research, there is no need for supplementing with antioxidants if your diet is complete. Excessive consumption can be injurious. So, all in all, it's probably okay if you take a supplement that includes these antioxidants, but be cautious not to overdo it.

Collagen Supplements

Let's recall what we covered briefly in chapter 1 regarding the most abundant form of protein in the body. As reported by Kerri-Ann Jennings, RN, in *Healthline* (2020):

> Collagen is key to the construction of cells, tissue, organs, and muscles, as well as being the 'glue 'that helps hold other protein molecules together. Over time, and through normal metabolic action, collagen becomes depleted, and this may occur with greater frequency among older men, as our bodies produce less collagen, and also lower quality collagen, that weakens as we age. You may see outwards signs of collagen deficiency in skin that is less supple, less firm.
>
> Certain bad habits can accelerate the decline of your collagen. These include intake of too many refined carbohydrates, especially sugar, too much sun exposure (which is also bad for your skin, drying it out, and potentially causing skin cancer), and smoking.
>
> You can **rebuild collagen through diet**, with vitamin C, and the amino acids proline and glycine, which are found in eggs, dairy,

fish, and meats. Nuts and seeds are good sources of the mineral copper, which also contributes to collagen regeneration. In general, rich, complete, natural sources of protein are ideal.

But what if your diet has not yet improved to include these essential foods, or you have not yet modified your behavior to avoid the sugars and refined carbohydrates, and excessive sun exposure, that acts negatively on collagen. That's where a collagen supplement comes in.

Studies on the value of collagen supplements are limited, but encouraging, showing that skin texture can improve, muscle mass may increase, and the pain of joint disorders like osteoarthritis may subside when supplements are taken.

There are two popular supplements to enhance collagen levels; both may be taken in pill form, or as a powder that may be mixed with foods or beverages:

> Gelatin, and hydrolyzed collagen. Each contains protein that is broken down into smaller peptides, and even smaller amino acids, which are easily assimilated and believed to be reconstituted as collagen where needed in the body.

Herbal supplements. This is one of the largest categories of supplements, and are based on extracts from plants. You may be familiar with ginseng, echinacea, ginkgo biloba, tea tree oil, among many others. Unlike prescription drugs and OTC medications, the U.S. The Food and Drug Administration (FDA) does not test, regulate or approve herbal supplements, or most other supplements, for that matter.

While the laboratories and companies that market supplements are legally responsible for product safety, the FDA does not verify safety or effectiveness, and does not verify that the claims, such as improved memory, enhanced masculinity, better sexual or physical performance, are true and clinically proven. Even the contents of the supplements may not be as listed.

When thinking about whether you need more of a vitamin or mineral, or need an antioxidant or other type of supplement, it is important to know how much of each nutrient you get from food and drinks, as well as from any supplements you take. Rather than guessing, the next time you visit your doctor or dietitian, tell them what supplements you are currently taking, and ask their opinion if you need to add any supplements to your diet. Seeking professional help will prevent you from taking too little, or too much.

Men's Health Forum" (2014, 2015) sums it up: A nutritionally complete diet precludes the need for supplements. All necessary vitamins and minerals will be contained in a diet with five fruits and five vegetables, nuts and seeds, legumes (beans), whole grains and fish, plus lean meat, in moderation.

However, if you are not prepared to follow a good diet, and tend to avoid vegetables and fresh fruits, are likely to eat prepared, processed foods, and don't get much sun exposure, then, yes, a daily supplement of vitamins and minerals is probably a good idea.

But if you take a supplement, **play it safe**; there is no benefit, and there can be potential harm, if you take excessive amounts, or mega-doses, of vitamins and minerals. Check the label and aim for amounts that supply 100% of the recommended daily amounts. At best, when you ingest too many vitamins and minerals, you are paying for the excess, which you'll be excreting in your urine.

If you check the labels of multivitamins, you may be astonished to read the amount of vitamin E to be almost 2,000% of the recommended allowance;

some of the B vitamins reaching as high as 4,000% the recommended allowance. A lower risk alternative is to select specific vitamins, like D, B6, B12, that you need, and take them individually, rather than in a 'shotgun 'multivitamin.

Testosterone

We'll complete this chapter with a subject that has the attention of most men once they are out of their forties.

It is directly associated, physically and in the mind, with masculinity, and with good reason. The male hormone testosterone is responsible for maintaining energy levels, keeping bones strong, maintaining muscle mass and, most notably, sustaining libido, or sexual interest and drive. It ensures genital sensitivity, virility, and high sperm count. There's no doubt of its importance, yet age causes testosterone gradually to decline. In addition to natural, age-related declines, poor diet and excessive alcohol consumption can further lower the levels.

The UK's National Health Service (NHS) reports that as men age, their testosterone declines by around 2% annually, beginning as early as age 35. According to the British Society for Sexual Medicine, symptoms of low testosterone, also called hypogonadism, include diminished libido and erectile dysfunction, as well as unexplained weight gain, depression and hot flashes. As reported by Siski Green in the UK health publication, 'Saga' (2017), at Edinburgh's Queen's Medical Research Institute, Richard Sharpe, a professor of human reproductive science, says that very low testosterone levels cause a reduced level of overall energy.

Is it possible to improve testosterone levels with a healthy diet that includes certain foods that are rich in nutrients? Health and wellbeing authority Daniel Coughlin, writing in 'Saga' (2017), lists foods that can help raise testosterone levels without medical supplements:

These include **oysters**, which supply zinc and vitamin D, and **fish**, since research correlates the omega-3 fatty acids and vitamin D in mackerel, salmon, sardines, anchovies and other cold-water fish with raising testosterone. Mackerel is also a good source of zinc.

Macadamia nuts are a good source of monounsaturated fats that are believed to raise testosterone, and the same can be said for extra virgin **olive oil,** a monounsaturated oil. A study conducted in Argentina confirms these findings, and separately, as you now know, monounsaturated olive oil is also good for cardiovascular health.

All nuts are considered beneficial, but in addition to macadamia nuts, **almonds** contain a range of vitamins and minerals, plus arginine, an amino acid that raises nitrate levels and can help reduce erectile dysfunction. **Honey** is also high in nitrates, and provides similar benefits; further, honey contains boron, an essential mineral, and the flavonoid chrysin, which maintains testosterone by blocking its conversion to estrogen.

Lean meat is recommended, since meat-eaters have higher levels of testosterone, and higher sperm counts, than vegetarians and vegans. For heart health, lean meats, like white meat chicken and turkey, are preferable to meats like beef with saturated fats.

Cruciferous vegetables, which include kale, cabbage, bok choy, cauliflower, and broccoli, are believed to raise testosterone levels and lower the female hormone estrogen, due to a molecule, indole-3-carbinol, which is found in this family of vegetables.

Eggs (which are now recommended, in moderation, as part of a heart-healthy diet), are high in complete protein, as well as vitamin D and calcium, all of which help sustain or raise testosterone levels.

Mushrooms contain phytochemicals that block an enzyme, aromatase, from increasing estrogen levels. Testing was conducted using popular button mushrooms. but the same results are probably associated with other forms of mushrooms.

Okay, we're ready now to move on to working a healthy diet into our lifestyle, putting what we've learned so far into practice.

Chapter 6: Healthy Eating in Practice

Knowing what you should be eating, and what to avoid, is a matter of knowledge and understanding. If a pop quiz were given to you today, especially in multiple-choice format, you could probably score pretty well (if you've been reading chapter-by-chapter to this point).

So, yes, you know more about healthy diets, but putting your knowledge into action is another thing. Can you improve your eating practices to enhance your health and manage your weight, without disrupting your life, and without having to count calories? Can a healthy diet be great tasting, composed of easy-to-find, and easy-to-prepare meals? Is it possible to eat healthy every day, not just on occasion?

The goal of this chapter is to lead you towards a modified lifestyle that you can embrace with enthusiasm, with a new perspective on how you are taking charge of your health, your body, your future wellbeing, and even your longevity. That's quite a promise, but it's achievable.

You're aware of the downsides of not following a healthy lifestyle with a healthy diet, so in the spirit of positivism, let's focus on the good side of the equation: reducing the risks of developing heart disease (or not aggravating it, if you already have some clogging in your arteries, or high blood pressure), preventing or diminishing type 2 diabetes, and other serious conditions, getting your weight down to normal, and helping to prevent digestive disorders, and increase regularity. Healthy eating may also help prevent some forms of cancer, and other diseases and conditions associated with an overactive immune system, that causes chronic inflammation and joint disorders. Just say to yourself, "Who needs it?" You're ready to take the path away from all those troubles.

Beyond improved health, upsides may include feeling better, and looking better, especially if there's extra weight and a potbelly to get rid of.

Your Individual Diet

You are an individual, and your personal preferences are to be treated with respect, to ensure that you can effectively transition to healthy dietary practices. Your individualism extends from what *foods you like*, to what *foods like you*; the foods that you are better able to digest and assimilate and turn to energy and rebuilding. You probably already know which foods give you indigestion, and force you to keep antacids handy. Chances are, those same irritating foods are among those not recommended for a healthy diet. Listen to your body, keep an open mind and be receptive to adopting a diet that will be healthy, and enjoyable.

Guidelines, Not Conformity

A study was reported in the "Journal of the American Medical Association" (2019), that concluded that diets that are **personalized to the individual** can be more effective that the one-diet-fits-all approach that has been traditionally relied upon. So you may want to think less about the standard food pyramid that the U.S. government has been advocating, and think more about what works best for you. (Below you'll find a completely new, healthy diet pyramid.)

You have a right to have your own personal tastes and preferences, and be assured that you should not have to follow a narrow, restrictive path of dietary choices, and can be free to make personal selections. No diet will be successful if it is disagreeable, or unpleasant, and it forces you to abandon everything you like.

But your individual preferences should still be within the recommended food groups, and should not include foods that have been identified as deleterious to your health, as well as your weight management. You may also find it easier to ease into the new lifestyle and diet, rather than abandoning things you are partial to. Just be aware that the sooner your diet is closer to ideal, the sooner your health and well-being will improve. There's more about resolution and transition to a healthy diet later in this chapter.

No two digestive systems are the same (imagine the varieties among billions of bacteria and other microbes that are unique to each person), so why should everyone follow the same diet? **Your gut bacteria are influential**, based on new findings that people chemically and biologically process foods differently, because of the unique composition of the complex bacterial microbiome in our guts.

The following section gets specific about dietary sensitivities, presents an ideal healthy diet you can embrace with enthusiasm, and helps with engaging and staying with your healthy diet.

Food Sensitivities

So it makes sense to know what foods agree with you, and especially, what foods do not. But medical examination of the microbiota relies on individual gut bacterial analysis, via stool samples, which is probably more than you want to submit to. A simple, but useful alternative, is to pay close attention to everything you eat, and try to identify anything that does not go down well for you. You'd be surprised to learn how sensitive you can be.

For example, if you feel bloated after eating a reasonable (not excessive) amount of wheat or rye-based bread, bagels, rolls, or pasta, you may have a gluten intolerance, and should try gluten-free products for a few weeks to see if the bloating or discomfort disappears.

Another common food-related disorder is lactose-intolerance; the inability to digest certain natural carbohydrates in milk, and other dairy products. If you suspect this may apply to you, based on gas, bloating, or pain after drinking milk, try switching to lactose-free milk, or one of the many non-dairy milk substitutes, based on soy, almonds, rice, or oats.

A more comprehensive test of dietary tolerance is called the FODMAP diet, which stands for foods that are "Fermentable Oligo-, Di-, Mono-saccharides And Polyols," which are short chain carbohydrates that are not well digested by your gut bacteria, and poorly absorbed in your small intestine. Symptoms include frequent bouts of gas, bloating, and stomach irritation. Chronic disorders with these conditions are irritable bowel syndrome (IBS) and Crohn's disease.

A diet that is low in FODMAP foods should only be considered a temporary plan, according to Hazel G. Veloso, a gastroenterologist at Johns Hopkins Medical Center. She says it's a short-term process "To determine which foods are troublesome." The idea is to initially eliminate all potentially disturbing foods, and once symptoms subside, gradually reintroduce foods to determine if they're okay, or not.

An exhaustive list of foods that are okay on a FODMAP diet, and foods that potentially are not well tolerated by your microbiome, has been compiled by a collaboration of Monash University in Melbourne, and King's College, London. If you suffer from IBS, Crohn's disease, or suspect you may have a number of food intolerances, including a condition called "Leaky Gut," enter "FODMAP" into a search bar, and you'll find quite a lot of information, including the foods to eat, and those to avoid. Not surprisingly, regular milk, and wheat and rye-containing foods are high on the FODMAP avoidance list. Yet most cheeses are okay, as is sourdough bread, since the questionable carbs have been pre-fermented, and are acceptable to the gut bacteria.

The Recommended Mediterranean Diet

It will come as no surprise, since the previous chapters have been hinting, that the **Mediterranean diet is the best dietary choice** for most of us, and is probably best for you. It's based on extensive experience, scientific study, and moreover, it is varied, giving you many choices of a wide diversity of healthy, great tasting foods.

Rated number one. "US News & World Report" evaluated 35 diets, and rated the Mediterranean diet number one overall. To be clear, this rating and recommendation is for all adults, male and female, but appears especially well-suited to men over 40, given the health concerns that arrive with age, Let's get into this diet's benefits and characteristics.

This diet first came into prominence when it was observed that people in countries bordering the Mediterranean, including Greece, Spain, Italy and southern France, live longer, are less prone to obesity, are healthier and less likely to have cardiovascular disease and cancer, or to develop type 2 diabetes. Yet they eat enthusiastically, and treat mealtime with a sense of pleasure every day.

No counting calories, but no junk foods, no processed foods either.

Importantly, in addition to eating a healthy diet, people of this region practice active lifestyles, which contributes to their overall wellbeing. Mostly by necessity, they are in motion, walking, climbing, bending, working; the opposite of being sedentary, and sitting all the time. (Chapter 7 will get you going, exercise-wise.)

Their diets may vary by nationality. The Greeks may eat differently than the French, for example, but their food selections have common characteristics:

> Mediterranean diets are based primarily on lots of vegetables and fruits, whole grains, nuts and seeds, fish and lean poultry, olive oil, and yes, red wine seems to be a common inclusion. What's missing: Meats loaded with saturated fats, and processed foods that are high in either sugar or salt, or both. Fried foods are minimal.

A **Mediterranean diet pyramid** was developed by the Harvard School of Public Health, in collaboration with the World Health Organization (WHO), and Boston-based Oldways, a nonprofit food and nutrition advisory service:

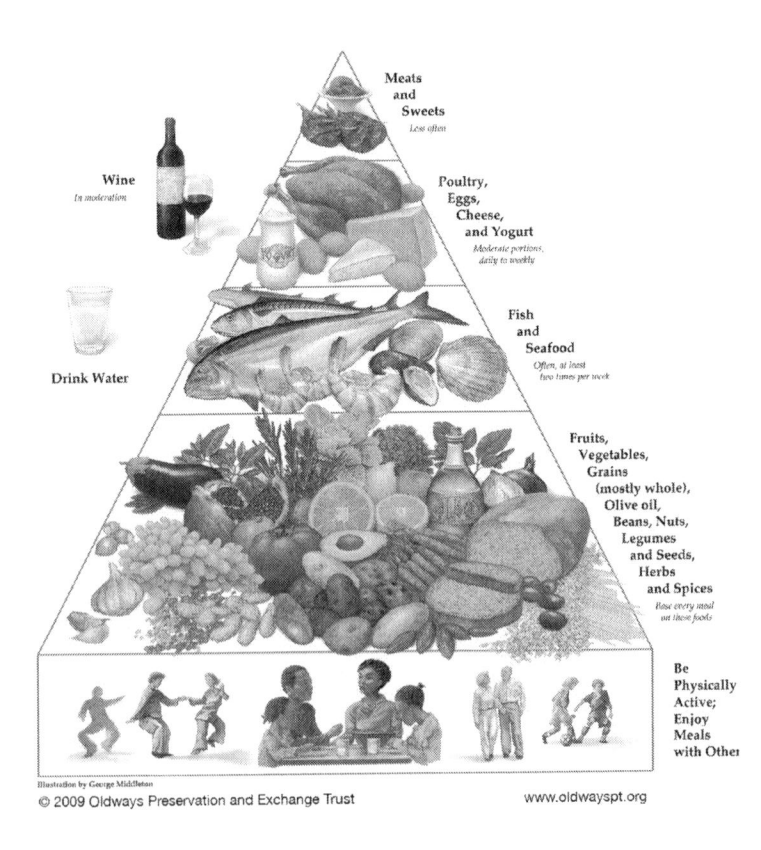

Starting from the bottom, just above the lifestyle images, level 2 is at the base of the food pyramid, with the foods that should form the largest part of your diet, and ending at the peak, level 5, the small tip of the pyramid.

130

- ❏ Base level **2**: *Everyday foods*, including whole grains, nuts and beans, vegetables in a profusion of variety and colors, healthy fats from olive oil, plus herbs and spices.
- ❏ Next level **3**: *Twice a week* servings of fish and seafood for healthy, complete protein, and beneficial omega-3 fatty acids.
- ❏ Next level **4**: *Several times per week* servings of eggs, dairy products (especially low-fat), and less frequently, lean cuts of poultry.
- ❏ Peak level **5**: *Occasional servings* of lean, unprocessed meats (which can include small portions of lean *red* meat), and sweets (other than fresh or dried fruits, which may be served daily).

Now, let's see how you can manageably adjust your daily eating routine to work with the recommended Mediterranean diet.

Planning for Special Dietary Goals

In addition to committing to a healthy diet, and assuming you are enthusiastic about the Mediterranean diet, you may have additional priorities, like weight loss, building muscle mass, and reducing hypertension.

Weight loss. Now that you are a middle age man, you may be finding weight loss more challenging than when you were young. That's because your metabolic rate is now slower, meaning your body is burning fewer calories per day. The obvious solution is to cut caloric intake, and the CDC recommends trying to ingest 500 fewer calories per day.

But if the idea is to not have to count calories...?

There are two key simple procedures to lose weight by cutting calories, yet without having to count calories: (1) reduce the sizes of portions, and (2) avoid fatty foods, fried foods, and foods high in sugar and refined carbohydrates, as well as all junk food. Eat responsibly in this manner, and the calorie reduction, and gradual weight loss, will occur automatically. Also, **eat out less often**. You will reduce calories, eat healthier, with lower fats, and sodium, you'll avoid dangerous trans fats, and you'll also save some money. Not a bad tradeoff.

More muscle mass. As testosterone declines, muscle mass declines, slowly, gradually, and fat can accumulate in place of muscle cells. Very simply, you'll need to increase the ratio of protein in your diet. But with a slower metabolism, you won't need as much protein as when you were younger. While the Mediterranean diet pyramid remains a reliable general guideline, you can *moderately* increase the fish, eggs, lean meat, plus beans, and protein rich soybean foods, including tofu, and natural edamame beans. Remember that meat and poultry protein sources can also contain saturated fats, so select lean cuts, and trim any visible fat.

High blood pressure. The Mayo Clinic (2020), and the National Institutes of Health are among the authorities recommending the **DASH** diet, or Dietary Approaches to Stop Hypertension, which aspires to lower systolic blood pressure by up to 14 points, by dietary changes, rather than medication. For a man with hypertension (systolic pressure of 130 or greater) who has not yet been following a healthy diet, adopting the Mediterranean diet will meet the DASH-encouraged emphasis on vegetables and fruits, nuts and seeds, whole grains, low fat dairy, fish instead of red meat, avoidance of processed meats and other processed foods.

But in addition, the DASH diet specifies limits on sodium: down from average 3,000 mg or more in typical American diets, to 2,300 mg, or if needed, 1,500 mg per day. It's important for the control of hypertension to be attentive to the sodium content of foods by reading the labels, and choosing the low sodium versions of canned and packaged foods. At the same time, cut back on the amount of salt you add during cooking and at mealtime.

Tip: Do not add salt while cooking. Instead, add a small amount of salt to the cooked food. This way, the salt will remain on the surface of the food, providing taste without having to saturate the food. Example: Don't add salt to the water you are boiling pasta in; just sprinkle a little salt once it's cooked.

Other dietary objectives, including reduction of **saturated fats**, are achievable with the Mediterranean diet. Elimination or steep reduction of fatty meats, saturated plant-derived and hydrogenated fats (like shortening) will go a long way in protecting heart health by preventing clogging of your arteries with plaque.

Avoidance of carbohydrates with a **high glycemic index** (which causes spikes in blood glucose and insulin) will also be a result of following the Mediterranean diet, which will replace refined carbohydrates and sugar-loaded foods with low glycemic index carbohydrates. including whole grains and seeds, vegetables and fruits. It will be important to avoid 'cheating 'so do not continue to snack on packaged junk foods, which are highly processed, and frequently loaded with sugar.

Same goes for pastries: Even pies, seemingly innocent with fruit filling, are high not only in added refined sugar, but the crust is loaded with saturated, hydrogenated fats from the shortening. For these reasons, most pies are very high in calories; this includes sweet pies, and also pot pies. If you can't resist, try not to eat too much of the crust.

Sticking With Your Healthy Diet

Agreeing with the concept of a healthy diet is one thing, but making it a fundamental component of your lifestyle can be challenging, especially after a lifetime of eating whatever you want. How do you give up the french fries, fried chicken, large servings of fatty meats, as well as avoiding donuts, and even ice cream, which contains large quantities of both sugar and saturated fats?

The answer is to resolve and commit, and also to shift gradually, less of a "cold turkey" approach, and more of a transition:

Resolution and transition. It's decision time. To successfully change your dietary practices and follow a new program of healthy eating, a personal commitment is needed. If you believe what we've covered so far, and feel you'd like to "buy in," the next step is to resolve to make it work for you. As mentioned, everything in the Mediterranean diet offers considerable flexibility and variety (you'll see recipe ideas in the last chapter), so you will have the latitude to select foods, and beverages that you like, or are willing to try.

You can transition into your healthy diet. There's no need to do a 180 degree turnaround on day one. Start with shifting from sugary cereals and snacks, and discover that whole grain cereals, breads and pastas are not only nutritious, but have far more flavor than foods with overprocessed, bleached flour and grains.

You may have not been caring for fish, for example, and are accustomed to grilled steak and hamburgers. You may be pleasantly surprised to discover that grilled salmon steak, perhaps with just a slight coating of butter, is amazingly flavorful and satisfying. Prefer burgers? Try a salmon burger, with a few flecks of cheese mixed in. Or, on the poultry side, most meat counters offer ground turkey (dark and white meat, or a combo), which form easily into burgers.

Exceptions. You will be faced with situations when your choices are limited, and you may have to make exceptions. Having **dinner as a guest** in someone's home, for example, means you may be subject to having to eat meat with saturated fats and fried foods, and have limited vegetable, salad and fruit options. Just be selective in what you choose to eat, cut away fat, remove fried food crust, and eat a bit less overall. Accept that exceptions will occur, and single episodes where you go "off diet," are okay, on occasion.

Another option is to call ahead and tell your host that you have some dietary restrictions, and if possible, could you have fish or chicken instead of beef, or beans instead of meat. People on vegetarian diets are accustomed to making these kinds of requests, and most hosts are understanding, when you give them a heads up.

When planning to eat out, before **selecting a restaurant,** go online to the restaurant's website and see the menu. Determine if the healthy meal choices are available and use that as a criterion of where to go for that meal occasion. In the restaurant, specify your preferences, especially if you are restricting salt.

For your starter course, get in the habit of ordering a mixed salad, and request the dressing (which can be high in calories) be served on the side, so you can limit how much you use. Starting with salad provides the *volumetric effect,* which helps fill you with low calorie nutrition, and reduces your appetite for the main course and dessert.

For the main course protein, a safe selection is grilled fish. For dessert, try to resist the cream and sugar-intensive desserts, and go for fresh fruit, if possible.

Intermittent Fasting

There are trends in diet management that involve fasting for a period each day, or fasting for several consecutive days. Most research on fasting has been conducted in laboratories with worms and mice; human research is limited. Those who advocate and practice fasting base its benefits on evolution, when our hunter/gatherer ancestors often went for long periods between meals. There are claims of increased longevity with fasting, but no quantitative clinical trials among humans to substantiate these claims.

Fasting for multiple days is not recommended without medical supervision, and may not be of interest to you, but you may consider easy-to-follow 16:8 intermittent fasting:

> You eat nothing for 16 hours, except drinking water to stay well hydrated. Then you eat the day's entire diet during the next 8 hours. Typically, the 8 hour eating cycle is the

middle of the day; 16 hours of fasting is from early evening through late morning. For example, eating from 10:00 AM to 6:00 PM, and fasting from 6:00 PM, through the night, and resuming eating at 10:00 AM the following morning. Alternatively, and more challenging, is to limit eating to 6 hours, and to fast for 18 hours.

Typically followers of intermittent fasting do not pay much attention to what they are eating—it is the fasting, not the food that counts for them—and there is no relevance to the Mediterranean diet, or any other heart-healthy diet. This is **not recommended.**

There is overwhelming evidence to confirm the effectiveness of the Mediterranean diet, and similar diets, in improving heart health, overall health, and increasing longevity, by rejecting saturated fats, refined carbohydrates and excessive sugar in foods and beverages, and focusing around vegetables and fruits, whole grains, cereals, and nuts, more fish and less meat, and olive oil instead of other fats, as we've been explaining. There is no such substantiating evidence for intermittent fasting without a healthy diet.

Is there value in combining a Mediterranean-type of diet with intermittent fasting? While there is no clinical verification that the fasting adds any benefits, as long as the diet is good, there is no harm in trying. Just remember to stay hydrated during the fasting period.

Let's close this chapter with the assurance that practical advice will be provided in chapter 8, including **recipes** for delicious, healthy meals that you can prepare with ease, without having to invest lots of time. As you will see, less is more in most cases, and simplicity triumphs over complexity. Full lists of ingredients you'll need to shop for, and easy-to-follow preparation and cooking instructions are included.

But first, on the following page is a suggested 7-day meal plan. It's based on easy-to-shop for, and easy to prepare Mediterranean diet recipes, all of which are provided in chapter 8.

The 7-day plan is a recommendation to get you started on what can become a life-long enjoyment of creating, preparing, and serving nutritious, delicious homemade meals.

7-Day Meal Plan

Shopping Guide (easy-to-find ingredients)

All ingredients for the recipes are listed with each recipe in Chapter 8. The lists are meant to be short, and based on what is readily available in any supermarket or well-stocked grocery. Your selections of the vegetables, fruits, fish, poultry and meats should be based on what's fresh, what looks good, and which are appealing to you. You will also find whole grains, cereals, nuts and olive oil in most markets. Shopping for healthy products can be confusing but it doesn't have to be. In order to make your shopping easier I suggest you to have a list of recommended products in your phone or to print it. To download your Mediterranean diet shopping list with tips how often to eat certain foods just go to link:

bit.ly/mediterraneanshopping

Be flexible, and be creative. Make variations based on your own ideas, and don't worry if an ingredient or two is hard to come by. Make substitutions that interest you.

Mediterranean Diet for Men: 7-Day Meal Plan

	Breakfast	Lunch	Dinner
Sunday 1,372 Calories	#1 Spicy Apple Oatmeal with Egg	#5 Chickpeas, Green Salad and Tuna	#12 Steamed Fish with Potatoes and Tomatoes
Monday 1,373 Calories	#2 Homemade Hot Muesli	#6 Grilled Salmon with Brown Rice	#13 Italian Meatballs and Spaghetti
Tuesday 1,424 Calories	#3 Overnight Oat Muesli	#7 Greek Chicken Salad	#14 Steamed Shrimp with Tomatoes and Pasta
Wednesday 1,480 Calories	#1 Spicy Apple Oatmeal with Egg	#8 Steamed Mussels with Quinoa	#15 Chicken Scaloppine Marsala Sauté with Polenta
Thursday 1,128 Calories	#2 Homemade Hot Muesli	#9 Vegetarian Split-Pea Soup	#16 Mediterranean Fish Stew
Friday 1,339 Calories	#3 Overnight Oat Muesli	#10 Fast Tuna Over Whole Grain Pasta	#17 Mediterranean Grilled Chicken over Spinach
Saturday 1,052 Calories	#4 Hearty Turkey Bacon and Eggs	#11 Split-Pea Soup (with meat)	#18 Steamed Seafood Mix with Tomatoes and Pasta

How many calories do you need? A mature man whose lifestyle is relatively inactive needs about 2,000 calories per day to maintain his current weight. If he has a moderately active lifestyle, 2,200 to 2,400 are needed, and a mature man who has an active lifestyle needs from 2,400 to 2,800 daily calories.

Meeting your daily calorie goals. As you can see in the table, the 3 meals per day do not meet the daily 2,000 or more calorie requirement for you - but that's to be expected, since your daily food and beverage intake will also include snacks, desserts, and beverages. Another way to meet your caloric and hunger needs is to increase the serving sizes, since what we have shown in the recipes you'll see in Chapter 8 are moderate-sized single servings. So, feel free to increase the recommended quantities, especially the meat and fish protein sources.

Serving Suggestions (start with a healthy salad)

Begin dinner meals with a mixed green salad, made with romaine or other lettuce, kale or spinach, tomatoes, green, or yellow peppers, and with a low calorie dressing, or a small amount of olive oil and balsamic vinegar. Dessert can be fresh fruit with low-fat yogurt.

Providing for Leftovers (big time saver)

Here's how to save time and get more for the same effort: Double the ingredients and serve half at dinner; reserve the 2nd half in a container and refrigerate up to one week. Or, freeze for longer storage. Reheat in the microwave.

Chapter 7 will bring you lifestyle tips, separate and apart from diet and nutrition, that will prepare you for maximum success.

Chapter 7: Lifestyle Tips for Maximum Success

A healthy lifestyle is made up of many elements, in addition to diet, including exercise routines to get into good cardiovascular condition, improving physical strength and flexibility. Your wellbeing also involves maintaining a healthy weight, managing stress, engaging in social interaction, keeping your mind engaged and challenged, and getting a good night's sleep, every night. Each of these elements interacts with the others, creating a synergistic effect.

The Benefits of Exercise

According to Web MD and other authorities, daily exercise is important for a range of health-related reasons. Cardiovascular exercise, which gets your heart pumping, and keeps it pumping, helps prevent the onset of heart disease and is beneficial to many other organs, including our brains.

The Cleveland Clinic (2020) states unequivocally that physical activity is the optimal method for men to improve heart health, increase muscular strength, balance, and flexibility. Even cognitive disorders, like dementia, can be prevented, or slowed in their onset and progression.

Weight management is a natural outcome of regular exercise, by raising your metabolic rate, and burning more calories per hour. Even after exercise is completed, your metabolic rate remains elevated, as your body works to restore and rebuild.

Ask your doctor. Caveat: Men who have been sedentary, and are ready to start an exercise program should check first with their doctor, just to make sure everything is okay. The doctor may be able to recommend specific exercise routines, and the intensity that is appropriate to your condition.

Exercise and fitness activities are categorized into two major groups: **cardiovascular**, and **resistance**. Each plays a key role in maintaining good health and improving longevity. A third category is **flexibility**, which may be achieved before and after the other major **exercises**, or by practicing yoga or pilates.

Cardiovascular exercise is also called aerobic exercise, because it involves increased oxygen supply through the heart and to all the major muscle groups, and is considered one of the most important ways to protect the heart, brain, and other organs. The Centers for Disease Control and Prevention (CDC) recommends we get a weekly total of 150 minutes of brisk walking, or other form of moderate intensity aerobic workout. This can be done by several longer sessions, or shorter daily walks, jogs or other forms of exercise, which can include swimming, elliptical machines and treadmills.

Ideally, **cardiovascular exercises** should be performed four or more days a week, and doing it daily makes it more of a habit, and easier to stay with. If you have not been doing cardio regularly (or at all), start slowly, with moderate speed and intensity. After a few weeks, you will be able to pick up the pace, increasing speed, and resistance if using an elliptical machine, or uphill, on a treadmill.

Benefits of walking. You can achieve good cardiovascular conditioning by walking at a comfortable but brisk pace for 20 minutes; try to do this every day. Remember that our prehistoric ancestors were continuously on the move, and this was mostly walking, not often running (except during rare occasions of hunting, or fleeing from danger).

Harvard Men's Health Watch (HMHW) scientists analyzed over 4,900 articles about the health benefits of walking. The consensus was that walking lowered the chances of heart disease by 31%, and reduced chances of dying during the 11 years of the study by 32%. There was a direct relationship between the amount of walking, the pace and the results. Greater benefits accrued to those who walked longer and faster. However, just walking a total of 5½ miles per week and at a slow 2 miles per hour, still measurably reduced the risks of heart disease. You do not need to strain or become breathless.

Other benefits of walking include minimal risks of injury, no need for lengthy warming up and cooling down, and you don't need to have special clothing or equipment, except for a good pair of walking shoes.

How much, how hard? If you are already engaged in aerobic exercise, and want to have a more qualitative workout, but are not sure how hard to go, these are the professional guidelines, which require less walking than the Harvard (HMHW) study, but encourage more intensity:

The UK Department of Health recommends that adults of all ages should be active every day, and perform a minimum of 2½ hours of moderate intensity cardiovascular exercise every week. If you work out five days a week for 30 minutes, you will achieve that level.

Walking, jogging, swimming, or other exercise at "moderate intensity" is a level where you are breathing deeply, and your pulse rate is elevated. Elevated means being at about 70% of your maximum aerobic capacity, based on your age. Here's how you can determine yours:

> Subtract your age from 220, and multiply it by 70%
>
> Age 30: 220 - 30 = 190 X 0.70 = 133 beats per minute
>
> Age 40: 220 - 40 = 180 X 0.70 = 126
>
> Age 50: 220 - 50 = 170 X 0.70 = 119
>
> Age 60: 220 - 60 = 160 X 0.70 = 112
>
> Age 70: 220 - 70 = 150 X 0.70 = 105

To measure your heart rate, count the beats you can feel in your neck or wrist for 10 seconds, then multiple by six.

It's evident that our "cruising speed" heart rate goes down as we age. Listen to your body, and if your pace of exercise seems uncomfortable, slow it down, and stay at a pace that feels okay. This is especially important when you are new to cardio exercise.

Your objective is to stay with it, and enjoy the experience, and not to burn out.

Resistance exercise is also important, so don't assume weight lifting is the exclusive domain of younger men. Here's why: Now that you are in your midlife, or beyond, you are losing bone mass, as well as muscle mass. You do not have to surrender to these conditions, because weight lifting, and using resistance machines in a health or fitness center (see below for resistance exercises at home) can keep you strong and solid. WebMD cites studies that men in their 50s who perform resistance exercises routinely can be as strong as men in their 20s, who do not.

Be careful to increase weights and resistance levels gradually. You're not as young as you once were, and while you can regain most, if not all of your previous strength, you need to get there progressively. As we get older, men should lift lighter weights, generally, and do more repetitions; that way, you can get a good workout without straining joints and ligaments.

Resistance exercises at home can be performed without any weights or equipment.

The following five exercises can be performed three to four times a week; you'll benefit from a day of recovery between sessions, so don't overdo it. Begin each session with slow stretching, reaching up, touching toes, twisting your trunk slowly in each direction, and whatever moves feel comfortable. Be sure not to strain or overextend.

1. **Pushups,** just as you probably did in your youth, are excellent to strengthen your core and abdominals, your shoulders, chest and arms. Start by doing a set of 10 repetitions (or fewer, if 10 is tough to start).

2. **Squats,** or deep-knee bends are great for your thighs. Stand with feet shoulder-width apart and slowly squat down until your thighs are parallel to the ground. Pause then rise to the upright position, pause, then repeat. If you have difficulty with your balance, keep one hand on a chair or dresser. Do 10 reps, if comfortable, or as many as you can without straining or overexerting.

3. **Crunches** will give your abdominals a good workout. Lay on your back, knees slightly raised while keeping your feet on the ground. and sit up about six inches. Hold for several seconds, then lower. Repeat 10 to 20 time, depending your ability. While in this position, you can do leg lifts, which are another way to strengthen your abs. Lying flat, raise you lets for several seconds, lower, and repeat.

4. **Jumping Jacks** will keep you on your toes and get your heart pumping, while giving your full legs a workout. Start with feet together, hands and sides, then hop each font about 10 inches to the side, as you swing your arms out and clap your hands over your head.

5. **Planks** are another core exercise, with additional benefits to shoulders and chest. There are two ways to do planks: assume the start position for the pushup, or, while lying flat, face down, rest on your forearms and push up. Hold the "up" position for up to 60 seconds, if you can. Just do this once and then continue to the next exercise.

Your objective is to keep moving; no pauses between each exercise. Once you have completed the "circuit" of five exercises, rest with light stretching for two minutes then repeat the sequence one more time, for a 2nd set. Finish by stretching again, to cool down.

Search online for demonstrations of these and other at-home resistance exercises, or you may join an **online exercise class**, with a trainer leading and advising.

Flexibility helps prevent injury, and will improve your overall mobility, balance, and ability to bend, turn, and, well, be flexible. **Yoga and pilates** are popular ways to become flexible and gain improved balance. Check online for demonstrations, and classes you can follow along. If you want better training and instruction, consider joining a yoga or pilates class close to where you live or work. Live classes offer the benefits of personal instruction, and the motivation and social interaction that comes in a group environment.

Another benefit of yoga, specifically, is the relaxation and focus through managed breathing, that accompanies the stretches and poses.

Meditation and Mindfulness

Men of your age have extensive life experience that has taught us valuable life lessons. We have assumed responsibilities, been productive and have made positive influences on situations. We've been through quite a lot, we know ourselves, and our families and friends have trust in our abilities and our character. Yet too often, our minds may be going off in the wrong direction, our ability to focus and concentrate may seem off track on occasion, and despite a healthy sense of self-esteem, we may find ourselves feeling tense or insecure.

This is where meditation and mindfulness come in. They are easy-to-practice ways to calm you, restore your sense of self, and help you achieve your full potential.

Meditation and mindfulness help you to think more clearly, to concentrate, to find inner peace and rebuild your self-esteem, and self-confidence, by focusing the mind and blocking or dismissing intruding thoughts. These simple techniques can relieve stress and help your immune system to function normally, and can help prevent anxiety and overreactions, and descent into bouts of depression. Practice meditation and mindfulness at your convenience, or whenever you need to calm down, refocus, or center yourself, and they will become valuable elements of your healthy lifestyle.

How to Meditate

There are many techniques, including well-known transcendental meditation, but here is a simple-to-use technique. It's called the *relaxation response*, and is good for those who prefer uncomplicated yet effective meditation. It was created following laboratory research by Dr. R. Benson, a physician who understood the positive effects of meditation, but wanted to avoid complicated mystiques.

The technique involves just sitting quietly, eyes closed, and being conscious of your breathing, every inhale and every exhale. Begin by inhaling deeply, then exhaling completely, and imagine 'one' silently, to yourself, while you exhale.

Continue this simple repetition of in-and-out deep breathing, and thinking 'one' on each full exhale, and you will find that it blocks outside thoughts from intruding.

Within a few minutes, the managed, deep breathing lowers stress, and activates the calming sympathetic nervous system. Beginners find relaxation response meditation easy to learn, and an instructor is not required.

Try to set aside 10 to 15 minutes at the same time every day to meditate, but you may also do it whenever you need a break from the stress of your work or other activities.

How to Practice Mindfulness

Mindfulness, or being in the moment, has been popularized because clinical studies have shown it's effective in lowering anxiety and stress, strengthening the immune system and preventing inflammation. It differs from meditation by not blocking all outside thoughts and impressions, but rather in using those stimuli to keep you focused on where you are and what's going on at that very moment. There's no thinking of the past, or the future, just the 'now. 'Mindfulness may be practiced at any time, anywhere, whereas meditation requires a quiet environment.

Here is a simple form of mindfulness we'll call *environmental discovery*. Whenever you feel stress or at any time, even if you are already calm, pause and place yourself in the now, the present. Pay attention and take note of where you are, and what you are doing at that very moment.

Sense and observe, using all of your senses. Listen and become aware of birds chirping, hear the voices of people, see trees, buildings, structures. Is there anything you can smell in the air, like newly cut grass, or fragrances of perfume, or the odors coming from the kitchen? Anything you can feel?

Let all of these discoveries and observations occupy your attention and keep odd, unrelated thoughts from intruding into your consciousness. To repeat, no thinking of the past or the future, only the present, the now.

Unlike meditation, which is more formal and structured, practicing mindfulness may be done whenever and wherever you need to regain your focus. By remaining aware of what you are doing, as you do it, you will take a greater interest and do a better job.

Mental Stimulation and Social Interaction

"**Use it or lose it,**" advises WebMD (2020) to men in their 60's and beyond, and it's in regard to slowing the onset of mental declines and cognitive disorders. We are encouraged to remain stimulated and mentally alert, by keeping our minds active and engaged. Our brain contains about 100 billion neurons, which make trillions of neural connections as we think, solve, interpret, remember, and experience. A healthy diet is important to help prevent the buildup of plaque and proteins that can interfere with the neural connections, but using the brain, challenging it, exercising it cognitively, are also important.

Do new things. You are encouraged to read, including a variety of subjects, to solve puzzles, and take challenging quizzes, adopt a new hobby or two, and even learn a new language. Or, at least try to learn some foreign language basics, like greetings and thank you, or how to count in different languages—these are easy ways to start learning a new language, and over time, as you gain confidence, these first steps can lead you to more expansive language learning.

Social interaction is another form of cognitive enrichment that is beneficial, and is based on engaging with other people. This includes more involvement with family and friends but can extend to people you don't normally speak with. Get in the habit of stopping to chat with people. An easy 'ice-breaker, 'or way to get someone to talk to you is to pay them a compliment, such as something they're wearing. If you approach someone walking a dog, you are almost guaranteed a friendly conversation if you ask about their dog.

In "13 Tips to Help Men Live Happier, Healthier and Longer Lives," Jonathan Caruthers, a health and wellness writer for the South Louisiana Medical Association (SLMA) (2020), recommends improving your relationships with friends, by going hiking or fishing, or eating out, or taking in a movie, and encouraging serious and challenging conversations that can deepen relationships.

Similarly, Carothers suggests improving your relationship with your spouse or life partner, by finding positive and encouraging things to say every day. This would seem to be of particular importance in long-term relationships, when couples may tend to take each other for granted.

The Benefits of Sleep

Sleep is a necessity for good health, and our need for sleep remains as we mature. Recent studies show that our brain is like a computer, needing to reboot and sort through the day's impressions and experiences. Phyllis Zee, Ph.D., professor of neurology and director of Northwestern University's Sleep Disorders Center, says in "Everyday Health" (2020), that a man in his midlife needs from seven to nine hours of sleep each night for full mental and physical health. Insufficient, regular sleep can lead to increased risks of obesity, diabetes, and other physical and emotional problems.

Here's why: Professor Zee says "Data show that with sleep loss, there are changes in the way the body handles glucose," that can cause prediabetic insulin resistance. Lack of sleep can also disrupt the regulation of appetite, causing you to overeat, and canceling out your dietary efforts to avoid becoming overweight or obese.

There are ways to optimize sleep, helping you to fall asleep, and stay asleep for a full restful night:

- ❏ Avoid coffee, tea and any other caffeine-rich beverages for six or more hours before sleep.

- Do not conduct any business or other potentially stressful activities for one hour before going to sleep.
- Log off your computer, and shut off your mobile phone, and silence the ringer at least 30 minutes before retiring; the glare of the screen is believed to prevent your adaptation to the night.
- Go to sleep and wake up at the same time every day; your sleep will improve with a consistent pattern.
- Do not use alcohol to help you to fall asleep. While it may provide immediate relaxation benefits, alcohol can interfere with the important dreaming cycle during the REM (rapid eye movement) sleep phase.
- Keep the room you sleep in dark, since your natural biorhythms react to light, and associate darkness with sleep. Also, keep the room cool and comfortable.
- You can help relax before sleep with a warm bath, or reading an interesting (not stressful) book or magazine. A light snack may help.
- When you find you can't fall asleep, don't worry about it. Briefly tense all of your muscles, then relax. Breathe deeply and

slowly, which can help bring about a meditative state.

❏ If you wake up during the night, which is common among men over 50 with enlarged prostates, keep the lights off while you use the toilet, and head right back to bed. Avoid anything that will cause you to further awaken.

Sleep and Your Immune System

Is it possible for your immune system, which protects you from infection and invading bacterial and viral pathogens, to be affected, positively or negatively, by your sleep behavior? The answer involves T cells, which are initiated by the adaptive immune system when the innate response, with white cells, is not sufficient, and the 'killer' T cells are needed. T cells attach to viruses and destroy their reproductive abilities, or simply chemically eradicate the viruses.

The Journal of Experimental Medicine reports on a study conducted by Dr. Stoyan Dimitro at the University of Tubingen in Germany among people able to sleep all night, and another group who could not sleep. Samples of blood samples from those who slept all night were compared to the group that remained awake all night.

Higher levels of T cell activation of integrin (which enables the T cells to adhere to viruses) was recorded among the good sleepers, indicating a positive relationship between the quality of sleep and the quality of the immune response. Dr. Dimitro believes that among the non-sleeping group, the effectiveness of the T cells was diminished by stress hormones, including adrenaline and norepinephrine.

Obviously, a strong immune response is crucial to health and longevity, since it makes the difference when it comes to protecting us from diseases, whether from bacteria that enter our bloodstream from a cut or injury, or from contaminated food, to viruses which invade our cells, take over the cells ' DNA, and use it to reproduce.

Okay, on to the last chapter, where we'll step into the kitchen and develop easy ways to plan menus, prepare and cook a range of delicious, healthy meals.

Chapter 8: Easy and Delicious Recipes for Your Optimal Health

Here are a number of recipes, based on the Mediterranean diet, that can get you well started on healthy breakfasts, lunches, and dinners. Each recipe is easy to follow, with simple preparation and short cooking times. As with any recipe, feel free to adjust, based on your preferences and the availability of ingredients. Be creative, and invent your own variations.

Bon appétit!

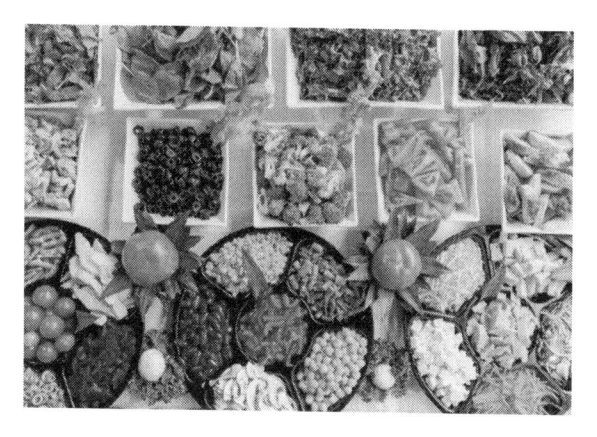

Breakfast Recipes

Breakfast Recipe #1- Spicy Apple Oatmeal with Egg

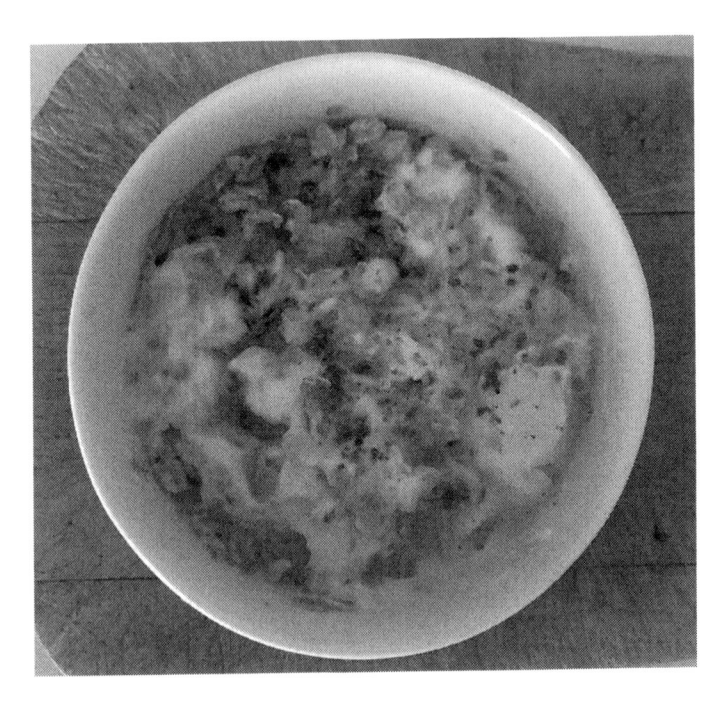

Servings: 1 adult
Preparation Time: 10 minutes
Cooking Time: 3 minutes

Recommended Ingredients

- 1/2 cup oatmeal (regular, not pre-cooked)
- 1/2 cup low fat or skim milk
- 1/2 medium-sized apple, chopped
- 1 large or extra-large egg, cage-free, and free range or pasture raised
- 1/4 tsp cinnamon powder
- 1/2 cup low fat Greek yogurt

Prepping and Cooking Directions

1. Mix milk and egg well in a microwaveable bowl until well blended.
2. Add oatmeal, apple, and cinnamon; stir well.
3. Place in the microwave oven and cook on high for 1 1/2 minutes.
4. Pause 20 seconds, then heat again on high for 1 1/2 minutes.
5. (Be attentive to prevent the mixture from boiling over top of bowl)
6. Remove from the microwave oven and carefully spoon into the serving bowl.
7. Spoon yogurt on top and lightly mix in.

Nutrition Facts for Spicy Apple Oatmeal with Egg:

Amount Per Serving

Calories 477.1

Total Fat 12.0 g

Saturated Fat 4.5 g

Polyunsaturated Fat 1.9 g

Monounsaturated Fat 4.0 g

Cholesterol 227.2 mg

Sodium 355.4 mg

Potassium 1,067.8 mg

Total Carbohydrate 69.4 g

Dietary Fiber 11.6 g

Sugars 32.4 g

Protein 27.5 g

Breakfast Recipe #2 - Homemade Hot Muesli

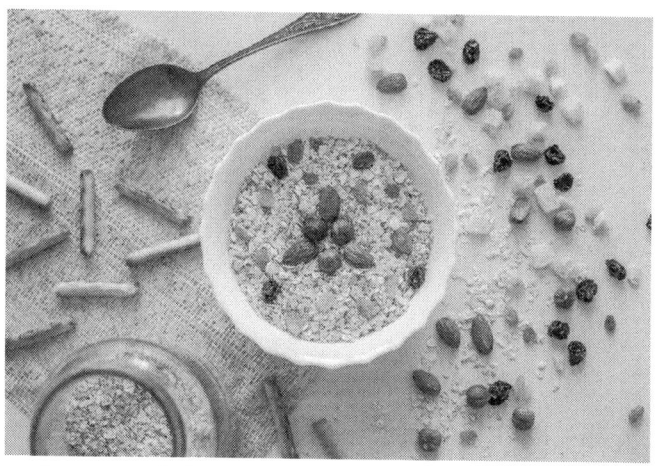

Servings: 1 adult
Preparation Time: 10 minutes
Cooking Time: 3 minutes

Recommended Ingredients

- ❏ 1/2 cup oatmeal (regular, not pre-cooked)
- ❏ 1/2 cup low fat or skim milk
- ❏ 1 tbsp unsalted nuts: peanuts, walnuts, pecans, almonds or mixed
- ❏ 1 tbsp flax seeds (optional)
- ❏ 4-6 prunes, chopped
- ❏ 1 tsp raisins
- ❏ 1/2 cup low fat Greek yogurt

Prepping and Cooking Directions

1. Mix milk, oatmeal. nuts, prunes, raisins, and flax seeds in a microwaveable bowl.
2. Place in the microwave oven and cook on high for 1 1/2 minutes.
3. Pause 20 seconds, then heat again on high for 1 minute. (Be attentive to prevent the mixture from boiling over top of bowl)
4. Remove from the microwave oven and spoon into the serving bowl, being careful since it is hot.
5. Spoon Greek yogurt on top and lightly mix in.

Nutrition Facts for Oatmeal Muesli:

Amount Per Serving

Calories 469.7

Sodium 402.2 mg

Total Fat 7.7 g

Potassium 1,117.9 mg

Saturated Fat 3.0 g

Total Carbohydrate 87.7 g

Polyunsaturated Fat 1.2 g

Dietary Fiber 6.2 g

Monounsaturated Fat 3.1 g

Sugars 48.0 g

Cholesterol 16.2 mg

Protein 23.9 g

Breakfast Recipe #3 - Overnight Oat Muesli

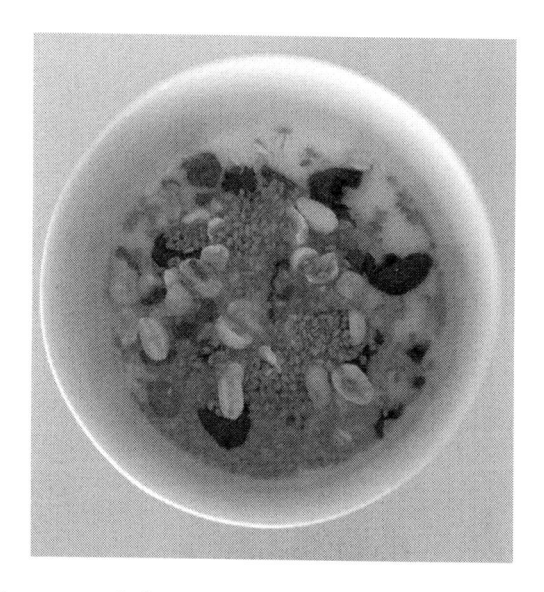

Servings: 1 adult
Preparation Time: 5 minutes
Cooking Time: none

Recommended Ingredients

- ❏ 1/2 cup oatmeal (regular, not pre-cooked)
- ❏ 1/3 cup low fat or skim milk
- ❏ 2 tbsp unsalted nuts: peanuts, walnuts, pecans, almonds or mixed
- ❏ 1 tbsp flax seeds (optional)
- ❏ 4-6 prunes, chopped
- ❏ 1 tsp raisins

Prepping Directions

1. Mix milk, oatmeal. nuts, prunes, raisins, and flax seeds in a bowl.
2. Cover and place in the refrigerator overnight.
3. Remove from the refrigerator 30 minutes before serving, if desired, to warm slightly.
4. If preferred to be eaten hot, place in the microwave for 45 seconds before serving.

Nutrition Facts for Overnight Muesli:

Amount Per Serving

Calories 469.7

Sodium 402.2 mg

Total Fat 7.7 g

Potassium 1,117.9 mg

Saturated Fat 3.0 g

Total Carbohydrate 87.7 g

Polyunsaturated Fat 1.2 g

Dietary Fiber 6.2 g

Monounsaturated Fat 3.1 g

Sugars 48.0 g

Cholesterol 16.2 mg

Protein 23.9 g

Breakfast Recipe #4 - Hearty Turkey Bacon and Eggs

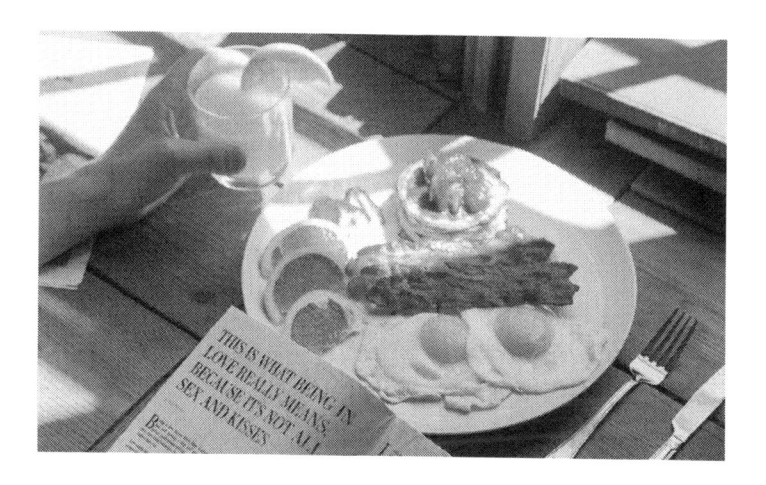

Servings: 1 adult
Preparation Time: 5 minutes
Cooking Time: 8-10 minutes

Recommended Ingredients

- ❏ 4 slices turkey bacon, minimally processed, natural, no preservatives
- ❏ 2 large or extra large eggs, cage-free, free range or pasture raised
- ❏ 1/2 tsp butter
- ❏ Salt and pepper to taste

Prepping and Cooking Directions

1. Place slices of turkey bacon in a skillet and heat over medium-hot burner
2. After 2 minutes, turn the slices and cook on the other side. After 1 minute, slide the slices to one side of the skillet, continuing to cook.
3. Immediately spread the butter on the open area of the skillet.
4. As soon as the butter starts to sizzle, carefully crack each eggshell and drop each egg onto the skillet.
5. Lower the heat if necessary, continue to cook the eggs until the whites are cooked.
6. If desired, use a spatula to flip the eggs, to cook briefly on the other side.
7. Use the spatula to lift the eggs and turkey bacon slices onto the plate.

Nutrition Facts for Hearty Turkey Bacon & Eggs:

Amount Per Serving

Calories 337.8

Total Fat 23.5 g

Saturated Fat 6.5 g

Polyunsaturated Fat 3.2 g

Monounsaturated Fat 6.6 g

Cholesterol 448.9 mg

Sodium 896.5 mg

Potassium 163.3 mg

Total Carbohydrate 2.0 g

Dietary Fiber 0.0 g

Sugars 1.7 g

Protein 36.2 g

Lunch Recipes

Lunch Recipe #5 - Chickpeas, Greens Salad & Tuna

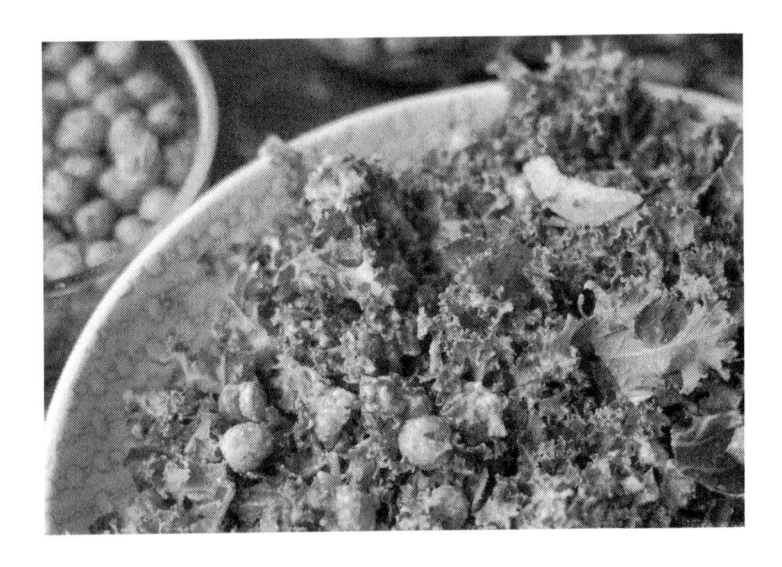

Servings: 2-3 adults
Preparation Time: 10 minutes
Cooking Time: None

Recommended Ingredients

- 1/2 can chickpeas (garbanzo beans), drained, rinsed
- 1 can tuna in water, drained
- 2 green onions (scallions), chopped
- 3-4 leaves of kale, cut into 1/2 inch-wide strips
- 6-8 leaves, romaine lettuce, cut into 1/2 inch-wide strips
- 2 tbsp chives, chopped
- 1/4 cup mint (optional)
- 1 tbsp olive oil (extra virgin)
- 1 tbsp balsamic vinegar, or apple cider vinegar
- 2 tsp dried herbs: thyme, rosemary, or oregano

Prepping Directions

1. Chop and slice leaves as directed above.
2. Drain tuna, separate into small chunks with fork.
3. Mix all ingredients in a large bowl.
4. May be served immediately, but will improve after a few hours in the refrigerator, so ideally prepare this dish earlier in the day.

Nutrition Facts for Chickpeas, Greens & Tuna:

Amount Per Serving

Calories 416.8	Sodium 688.4 mg
Total Fat 16.7 g	Potassium 801.7 mg
Saturated Fat 3.0 g	Total Carbohydrate 39.0 g
Polyunsaturated Fat 2.6 g	Dietary Fiber 7.3 g
Monounsaturated Fat 10.3 g	Sugars 0.7 g
Cholesterol 40.0 mg	**Protein 31.2 g**

Lunch Recipe # 6 - Grilled Salmon with Brown Rice

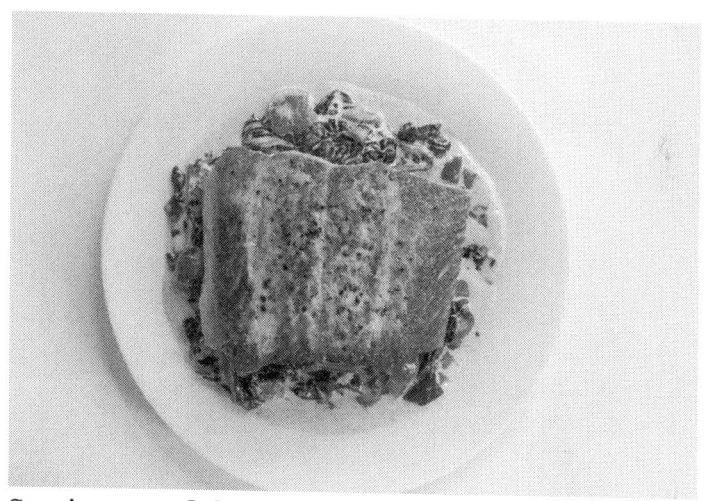

Servings: 2 adults
Preparation Time: 10 minutes
Cooking Time: 20 minutes

Recommended Ingredients

- 12 oz salmon steak, (Coho, Sockeye, Atlantic or Pacific (6 oz serving per person)
- Pinch of grey sea salt, to taste (optional for salt-free diets)
- 7/8 cup brown rice, or brown rice-wild rice mixture.
- 1/2 tsp butter (optional)

Cooking Directions

1. Bring 2 cups of water to a boil in a small saucepan or pot, with a lid or cover.
2. Add the rice, and turn down the heat to simmer. Cover the pot.
3. Turn on the oven to grill and preheat. Place the grill in a medium high position.
4. Keep an eye on the rice to make sure it keeps simmering.
5. Cover an oven-proof pan or cookie sheet with a sheet of aluminum foil.
6. Slightly butter the foil by rubbing lightly with the butter stick while cold.
7. Place the salmon steak directly on the foil and put in the oven.
8. As soon as the rice has absorbed all, or almost all the water, turn off the heat, but keep covered. If adding butter, do so now, stir well.
9. Check the salmon to make sure it's not burning, and remove from the oven after 15 minutes. The grilling is on one side only.
10. Place half the salmon steak on each plate, with half the rice. Serve immediately. If desired, a pinch or two of salt may be sprinkled over the salmon and rice.

Nutrition Facts for Salmon with Brown rice:

Amount Per Serving

Calories 411.1

Total Fat 15.9 g

Saturated Fat 4.4 g

Polyunsaturated Fat 4.9 g

Monounsaturated Fat 5.0 g

Cholesterol 104.9 mg

Sodium 108.8 mg

Potassium 884.8 mg

Total Carbohydrate 27.6 g

Dietary Fiber 2.2 g

Sugars 0.3 g

Protein 36.9 g

Lunch Recipe #7 - Greek Chicken Salad

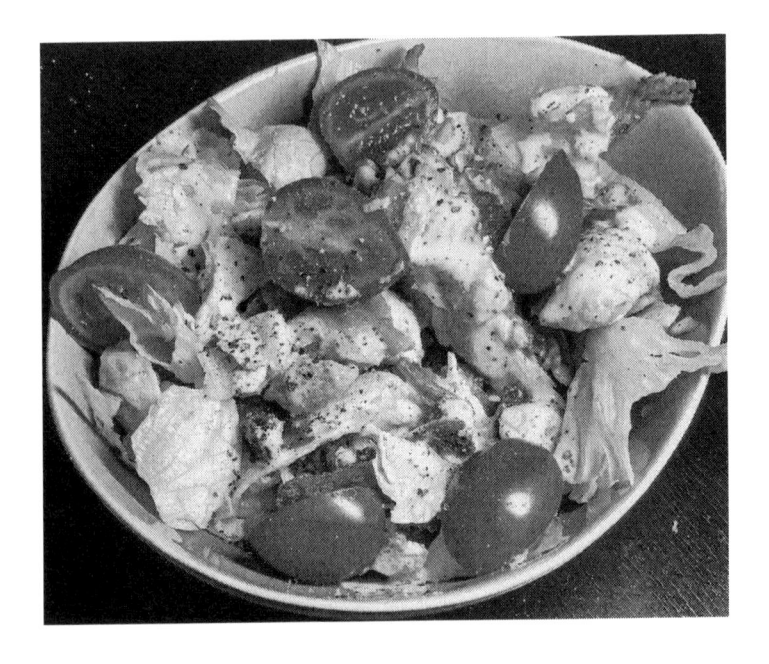

Servings: 2 adults
Preparation Time: 10-15 minutes
Cooking Time: none (after overnight soak)

Recommended Ingredients

- 2 cups white meat chicken, cooked and cubed
- 1 small onion, cubed
- 2 medium-large tomatoes, sliced
- 1 cup green, red and yellow peppers, chopped
- 2 tbsp olive oil (extra virgin)
- 1/3 tsp oregano
- 2 stalks green onions (scallions), chopped
- 1/4 cup fresh basil leaves
- 3-4 romaine lettuce leaves, uncut
- 3/4 cup feta cheese, cut into 1/2 inch cubes
- 8-10 Greek Kalamata olives, pitted

Prepping and Cooking Directions

1. Combine all ingredients except romaine lettuce leaves and feta cheese in a large bowl, and stir to mix well. Ensure tha ingredients are lightly coated with olive oil.
2. Add the feta cheese cubes and gently stir to mix with other ingredients.
3. Arrange 2 romaine leaves on each plate.
4. Spoon mixture of ingredients over the romaine leaves, to serve.

Nutrition Facts for Greek Chicken Salad:

Amount Per Serving

Calories 488.4

Sodium 641.5 mg

Total Fat 26.8 g

Potassium 781.2 mg

Saturated Fat 7.7 g

Total Carbohydrate 18.0 g

Polyunsaturated Fat 3.0 g

Dietary Fiber 4.2 g

Monounsaturated Fat 14.1 g

Sugars 8.0 g

Cholesterol 130.6 mg

Protein 45.4 g

Lunch Recipe #8 - Steamed Mussels with Quinoa

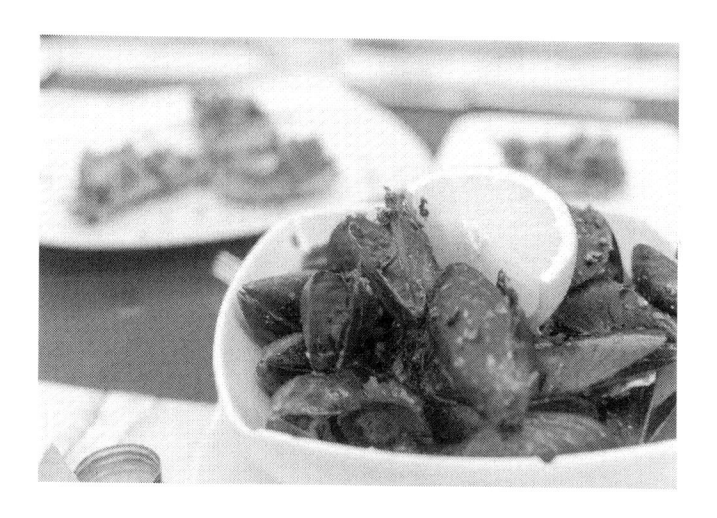

Servings: 2 adults
Preparation Time: 10-15 minutes
Cooking Time: 10 minutes

Recommended Ingredients

- 1 pound mussels, soak in cool water, drained and rinsed
- 1 onion, finely chopped
- 1/4 cup celery, finely chopped
- 1 tsp dried basil or 1/4 cup fresh basil, chopped
- 1 bay leaf (optional)
- 1 tbsp olive oil (extra virgin)
- 1/2 cup white wine, or vermouth
- Fresh parsley or cilantro, chopped
- 1 1/2 cups quinoa, previously cooked, and warm

Prepping and Cooking Directions

1. Drain the mussels and pat dry with paper towels. Pull any beards (threads or strands coming out the shells). Discard any mussels that are broken, or wide open.
2. Combine all ingredients except mussels, wine, and parsley in a large cooking pot and stir, turning heat to medium-high.

3. Sauté and as soon as the mixture is soft, add the wine, and mussels, and turn the heat up to high. Cover the pot.
4. Once steam starts to emerge from the pot, turn down the heat. Leave to simmer for another minute while spooning the quinoa into large serving bowls.
5. Using a large spatula or a cup, scoop up the mussels and pour over the quinoa. Be sure to tip the pot to collect the liquid, which should be poured over the mussels.
6. Serve with parsley or cilantro sprinkled over everything.

Nutrition Facts for Mussels with Quinoa:

Amount Per Serving

Calories 563.9

Sodium 479.9 mg

Total Fat 22.1 g

Potassium 644.5 mg

Saturated Fat 3.0 g

Total Carbohydrate 48.2 g

Polyunsaturated Fat 3.0 g

Dietary Fiber 5.3 g

Monounsaturated Fat 11.2 g

Sugars 7.4 g

Cholesterol 63.5 mg

Protein 34.3 g

Lunch Recipe #9 - Vegetarian Split Pea Soup

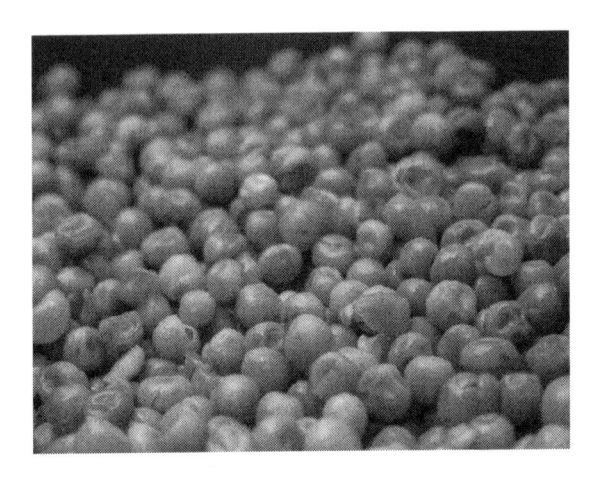

Servings: 2 adults
Preparation Time: 10 minutes
Cooking Time: 40 minutes (after overnight soak)

Recommended Ingredients

- ❏ 1 cup dried split peas
- ❏ 1/2 cup fresh or frozen green peas
- ❏ 2 carrots, or 12 mini carrots, sliced
- ❏ 1 onion, chopped.
- ❏ 2 stalks celery, chopped
- ❏ 3 cups water (or vegetable stock)
- ❏ 1/2 cup low fat Greek yogurt (optional)

Prepping and Cooking Directions

1. Place the split peas and water (or vegetable stock) into a cooking pot the night before, and allow to soak overnight. (This greatly reduces cooking time.)
2. 40 minutes before serving, turn on a cooktop burner to medium-high heat.
3. Add the sliced carrots, onion, celery, and fresh peas to the cooking pot.
4. Bring to a boil, then lower the heat to simmer, and cover the pot.
5. Check and stir frequently to make sure the soup is not sticking to the bottom of the pot or burning.
6. Serve with whole grain bread, lightly toasted.
7. When serving, spoon 1/4 cup Greek yogurt on top of each bowl and lightly mix in. (Optional: Without yogurt, this recipe is okay for vegans)

Nutrition Facts for Split-Pea Soup:

Amount Per Serving

Calories 203.8

Total Fat 0.8 g

Saturated Fat 0.1 g

Polyunsaturated Fat 0.4 g

Monounsaturated Fat 0.1 g

Cholesterol 0.0 mg

Sodium 134.6 mg

Potassium 842.7 mg

Total Carbohydrate 39.1 g

Dietary Fiber 13.5 g

Sugars 10.7 g

Protein 12.3 g

Lunch Recipe # 10 - Fast Tuna Over Whole Grain Pasta

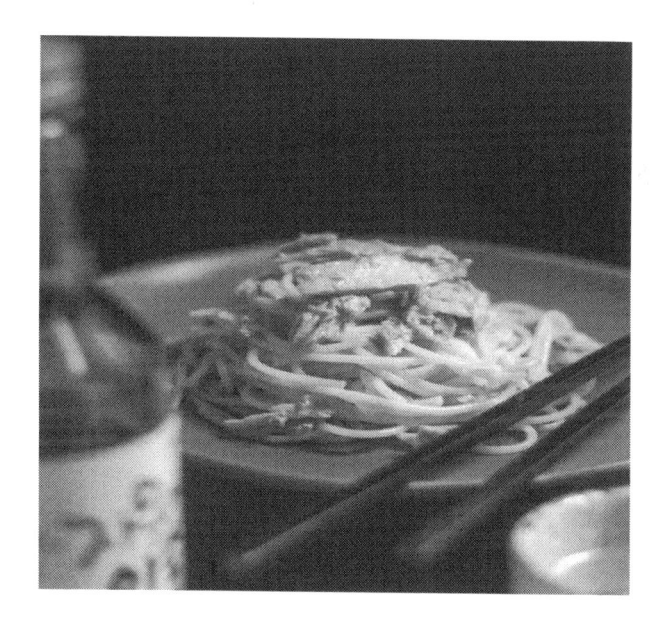

Servings: 2 adults
Preparation Time: 6 minutes
Cooking Time: 20 minutes

Recommended Ingredients

- One 5 oz can, tuna in olive oil. (Do not drain oil)
- 1/2 can Italian-style chopped or diced tomatoes
- 8 black olives, pitted, halved
- Pinch of grey sea salt, to taste (optional for salt-free diets)
- Ground black pepper, to taste
- 3/4 tsp oregano or thyme
- Bunch cilantro or parsley, chopped.
- Grated parmesan cheese
- 1/3 lb dried whole wheat spaghetti (or other whole grain pasta)

Prepping and Cooking Directions

1. Boil the pasta for 7-8 minutes or according to directions on the box.
2. While pasta is cooking, place all ingredients except cheese in a microwaveable container, stir well to mix in the tuna, and cook on high setting for 2 minutes. Cover to prevent splattering.

3. When the pasta is al-dente (cooked, with slight firmness, not soggy), drain and use a fork to remove a serving to each plate.
4. Give the tuna mixture an additional 30 seconds on high in the microwave.
5. Carefully remove the container, lift lid, being careful of steam, and spoon mixture over the pasta.
6. Sprinkle the parmesan cheese over the mixture and pasta.

Nutrition Facts for Tuna with Pasta:

Amount Per Serving

Calories 417.9	Sodium 495.7 mg
Total Fat 11.3 g	Potassium 539.2 mg
Saturated Fat 2.7 g	Total Carbohydrate 46.0 g
Polyunsaturated Fat 3.1 g	Dietary Fiber 8.8 g
Monounsaturated Fat 4.4 g	Sugars 5.5 g
Cholesterol 19.3 mg	**Protein 36.3 g**

Lunch Recipe #11 - Split Pea Soup (with meat)

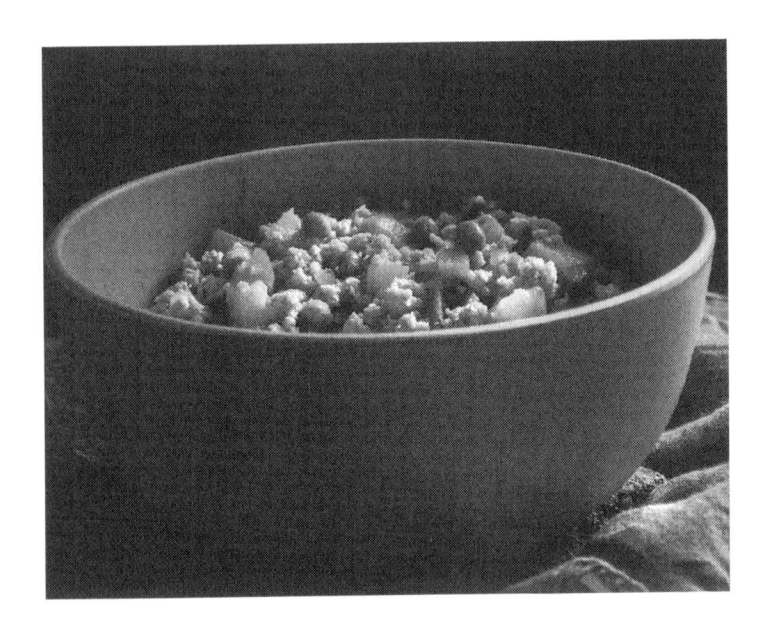

Servings: 2 adults
Preparation Time: 10 minutes
Cooking Time: 40 minutes (after overnight soak)
Follow **Lunch Recipe #9** and add:

- 1 cup lean ham, turkey, or chicken, cut into cubes
- 3 cups beef or chicken stock, or water

Nutrition Facts for Split-Pea Soup with Meat:

Amount Per Serving

Calories 248.8

Total Fat 2.8 g

Saturated Fat 0.8 g

Polyunsaturated Fat 0.9 g

Monounsaturated Fat 0.5 g

Cholesterol 48.3 mg

Sodium 153.6 mg

Potassium 844.7 mg

Total Carbohydrate 27.2 g

Dietary Fiber 9.2 g

Sugars 8.2 g

Protein 28.9 g

Dinner Recipes

Dinner Recipe #12 - Steamed Fish with Potatoes and Tomatoes

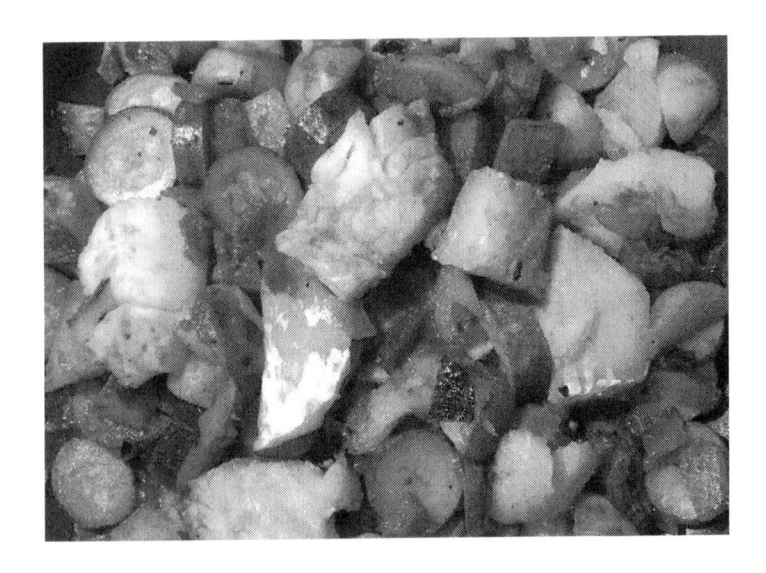

Servings: 2 adults
Preparation Time: 10 minutes
Cooking Time: 20 minutes

Recommended Ingredients

- 3 small potatoes, unpeeled, sliced
- 2 medium tomatoes, sliced (or 12 cherry tomatoes, halved)
- 8 black or green olives, pitted, halved (optional for salt-free diets)
- 1 tbsp olive oil (extra virgin)
- 1 small onion, diced
- 12-14 oz cod, for other white fish, like haddock halibut, 6-7 oz piece per person
- Pinch of grey sea salt, to taste (optional for salt-free diets)
- Ground black pepper
- Squeeze of lemon juice
- White wine, 1/4 cup

Prepping and Cooking Directions

1. Turn on the oven and preheat to 385 °F.
2. Spread out a large sheet of aluminum foil.
3. Spread out the sliced potatoes on the right half side of the foil.
4. Put the tomatoes, olives, lemon juice, wine, salt and pepper in a bowl and stir until blended.

5. Carefully lift the cod or other fish and arrange on top of the sliced potatoes.
6. Now carefully pour the tomato-based mixture on top of the fish.
7. Fold the left half of the foil over the fish, potatoes and tomato mixture, so that it is fully covered by the foil.
8. Carefully pinch or fold all the edges of the foil to create a tight seal.
9. Check to ensure that all sides of the foil are sealed, so no steam or mixture can leak.
10. Put the sealed foil package on a baking sheet or in a large enough pan.
11. Put the sheet or pan in the oven, and cook for about 20 minutes.
12. Carefully remove the pan or baking sheet from the oven, and use scissors to cut open the foil to reveal the contents.
13. Using a spatula, place one piece of fish on each plate, and spoon the potato and tomato mixture on top of the fish. It may help to have a large spoon to scoop up the wet ingredients.

Nutrition Facts for Steamed. Fish, Potatoes & Tomatoes:

Amount Per Serving

Calories 486.4

Sodium 417.6 mg

Total Fat 10.6 g

Potassium 1,531.2 mg

Saturated Fat 1.6 g

Total Carbohydrate 42.1 g

Polyunsaturated Fat 1.5 g

Dietary Fiber 7.2 g

Monounsaturated Fat 6.5 g

Sugars 5.0 g

Cholesterol 109.2 mg

Protein 49.2 g

Dinner Recipe #13 - Italian Meatballs and Spaghetti

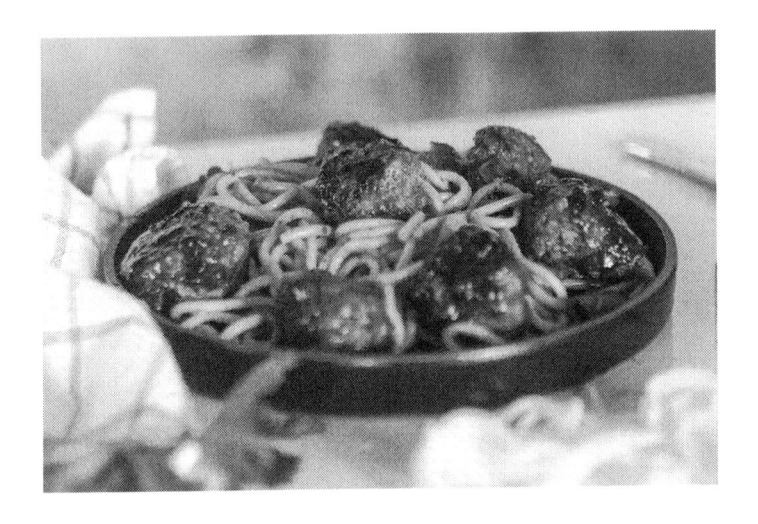

Servings: 2 adults
Preparation Time: 10 minutes
Cooking Time: 30 minutes

Recommended Ingredients

- 3/4 lb lean (10% fat or less) ground beef, or ground turkey
- 1/2 can Italian-style chopped or diced tomatoes
- 4 black or green olives, pitted, halved
- 1 medium onion, diced
- ½ tbsp olive oil (extra virgin)
- Pinch of grey sea salt, to taste (optional for salt-free diets)
- Ground black pepper
- 3/4 tsp oregano
- Bunch cilantro, chopped.
- 2-3 leaves kale, chopped (optional)
- White wine, 1/4 cup
- 1/3 lb dried whole wheat spaghetti (or other whole grain pasta)

Prepping and Cooking Directions

1. Turn on the oven and preheat to 400 °F.
2. Spread out a large sheet of aluminum foil.
3. Divide the meat into 12 to 14 equal chunks and roll into balls.
4. Place the meatballs on the right half side of the foil.
5. Put the chopped/diced tomatoes, olives, wine, salt and pepper, oregano in a bowl and stir until blended.
6. Now carefully pour the tomato-based mixture on top of the meatballs.
7. Fold the left half of the foil over the meatballs and tomato mixture.
8. Carefully pinch or fold all the edges of the foil to create a tight seal.
9. Check to ensure that all sides of the foil are sealed, so no steam can leak out.
10. Put the sealed foil package on a baking sheet or in a large enough pan.
11. Put the sheet or pan in the oven, and cook for about 30 minutes.
12. Boil the pasta for 7-8 minutes or according to directions on box.
13. When the pasta is al-dente (cooked, with slight firmness, not soggy), drain and use a fork to remove a serving to each plate.

14. Carefully remove the pan or baking sheet from the oven, and cut open the foil.
15. Using a large spoon, place half the meatballs, and half the tomato mixture on top of the pasta on each plate.

Nutrition Facts for Spaghetti with Meatballs:

Amount Per Serving

Calories 492.0

Total Fat 21.3 g

Saturated Fat 5.1 g

Polyunsaturated Fat 1.1 g

Monounsaturated Fat 6.3 g

Cholesterol 120.0 mg

Sodium 375.2 mg

Potassium 352.7 mg

Total Carbohydrate 34.2 g

Dietary Fiber 6.3 g

Sugars 3.9 g

Protein 39.8 g

Dinner Recipe #14 - Steamed Shrimp with Tomatoes and Pasta

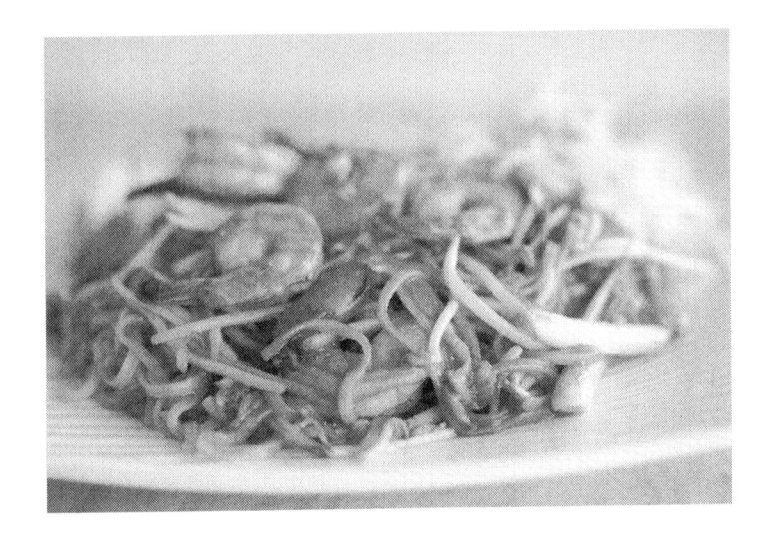

Servings: 2 adults
Preparation Time: 10 minutes
Cooking Time: 20 minutes

Recommended Ingredients

- 1 lb shrimp, either regular size or jumbo, fresh or frozen
- 2 medium tomatoes, sliced (or 12 cherry tomatoes, halved)
- 8 black or green olives, pitted, halved (optional for salt-free diets)
- ½ tbsp olive oil (extra virgin)
- 3-4 anchovies (optional for salt-free diets)
- Pinch of grey sea salt, to taste (optional for salt-free diets)
- Ground black pepper
- 1/2 tsp oregano
- White wine, 1/4 cup
- 1/3 lb whole wheat spaghetti or linguine,

Prepping and Cooking Directions: Same as for **Dinner Recipe #12,** but serve over pasta, simmered for 7-8 minutes until al-dente (cooked, with slight firmness, not soggy).

Nutrition Facts for Shrimp with Tomatoes & Pasta:

Amount Per Serving

Calories 465.7

Total Fat 13.9 g

Saturated Fat 2.2 g

Polyunsaturated Fat 2.8 g

Monounsaturated Fat 7.2 g

Cholesterol 351.3 mg

Sodium 858.3 mg

Potassium 570.1 mg

Total Carbohydrate 26.9 g

Dietary Fiber 4.6 g

Sugars 0.9 g

Protein 53.3 g

Dinner Recipe #15 - Chicken Scaloppine Marsala Sauté with Polenta

Servings: 2 adults
Preparation Time: 10 minutes
Cooking Time: 20 minutes

Recommended Ingredients

- ❏ 1 lb (or less) chicken breast, sliced horizontally to thin pieces
- ❏ 6 - 8 large brown mushrooms (or 12 small/medium)
- ❏ Whole grain flour (wheat, rye, spelt, or rice)
- ❏ 1/2 cup sweet marsala (dry also okay)
- ❏ 1/2 onion, sliced
- ❏ 1 tbsp olive oil (extra virgin)
- ❏ 6 slices polenta

Prepping and Cooking Directions

1. Warm a pan or skillet on the cooktop, medium heat.
2. Slice the onion and mushrooms.
3. Place the onions and mushrooms in the skillet with the olive oil

4. Sauté the onions and mushrooms, until they start to brown
5. Meanwhile, spread out the sliced chicken and cut into 6 pieces.
6. Lightly flour one side, turn and flour the other side.
7. Push the onions and mushrooms to the sides of the pan.
8. Add the slices of chicken and brown on one side.
9. Turn the chicken and brown on the other side.
10. Turn up heat and add marsala, bring to a boil.
11. Reduce heat and simmer until marsala is reduced by half.
12. Add the polenta, and stir.
13. Cover and turn down heat, simmer for 2 minutes.
14. Using a spatula, lift chicken to plates; use a large spoon to remove the pieces of polenta and sauce.

Nutrition Facts for Chicken Scaloppine with Polenta:

Amount Per Serving

Calories 444.5

Total Fat 10.7 g

Saturated Fat 1.9 g

Polyunsaturated Fat 1.7 g

Monounsaturated Fat 6.0 g

Cholesterol 70.2 mg

Sodium 531.8 mg

Potassium 657.7 mg

Total Carbohydrate 49.0 g

Dietary Fiber 6.8 g

Sugars 6.5 g

Protein 34.1 g

Dinner Recipe #16 - Mediterranean Fish Stew

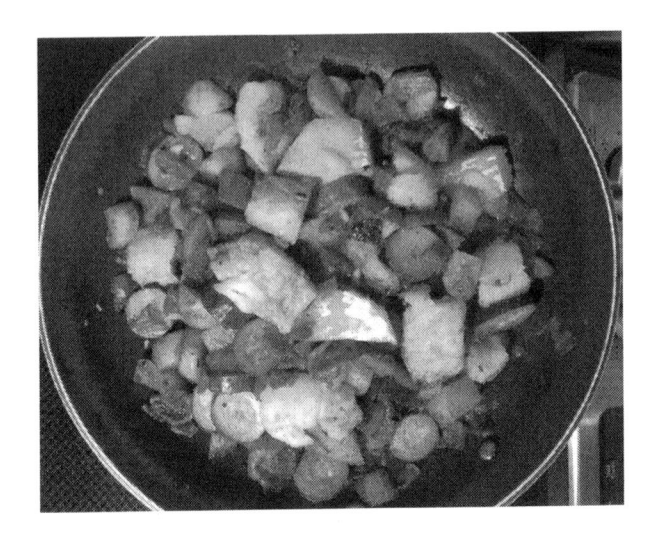

Servings: 2 adults
Preparation Time: 20 minutes
Cooking Time: 20 minutes

Recommended Ingredients

- 3/4 to 7/8 lb white fish, ideally cod or halibut or haddock
- 2 medium tomatoes or 1/2 can chopped tomatoes
- 1 small onion, or 1/2 large onion, diced
- 1 small green zucchini, sliced 1/4 inch thick
- 1 small yellow squash, sliced 1/4 inch thick
- 2-3 bay leaves
- 1 tsp oregano
- 2 tbsp olive oil (extra virgin)
- 1/4 cup vermouth or other white wine
- 1/2 tsp grey sea salt (optional)
- 1/4 tsp ground pepper, to taste

Prepping and Cooking Directions

1. Warm a pan or large skillet on the cooktop, medium heat.
2. Slice the onion, and place in the skillet with the olive oil.
3. Sauté the onions until they start to brown.
4. Slice the zucchini and squash while onions are browning, add to skillet and stir.

5. Add the tomatoes (fresh or canned) and stir mixture.
6. Lower the heat and cover the skillet, leave to simmer.
7. Cut the white fish into 1-inch cubes and add to the mixture in skillet, cover, simmer on low heat for 10 minutes.
8. Use a large spoon, or a cup, to serve stew into bowls, being sure to fairly divide the mixture and the liquid.

Nutrition Facts for Mediterranean Fish Stew

Amount Per Serving

Calories 454.6

Total Fat 16.5 g

Saturated Fat 2.4 g

Polyunsaturated Fat 2.4 g

Monounsaturated Fat 10.3 g

Cholesterol 93.6 mg

Sodium 299.0 mg

Potassium 2,071.2 mg

Total Carbohydrate 28.0 g

Dietary Fiber 8.1 g

Sugars 16.9 g

Protein 45.6 g

Dinner Recipe #17 - Mediterranean Grilled Chicken over Spinach

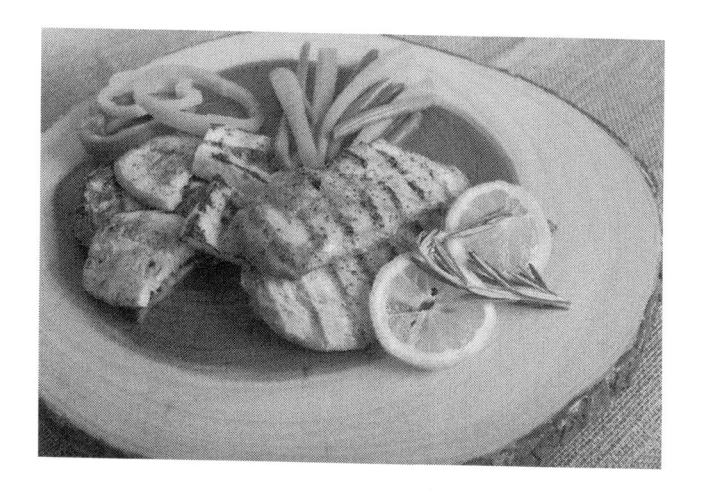

Servings: 2 adults
Preparation Time: 20 minutes
Cooking Time: 20 minutes

Recommended Ingredients

- 2 skinless and boneless chicken breasts or filets, each 6 oz
- 1 14 oz can chopped or diced tomatoes (fire-roasted if available)
- 1 cup baby spinach leaves
- 6-8 kalamata olives, pitted
- 1 tbsp olive oil (extra virgin) for chicken
- 1 tbsp olive oil (extra virgin) for tomatoes
- 1/8 cup vermouth or other white wine
- 1/4 tsp grey sea salt (optional)
- 1/4 tsp ground pepper, to taste
- 1/3 cup feta cheese, crumbled or finely chopped

Prepping and Cooking Directions

1. Warm a pan or large skillet on the cooktop, high heat.
2. Coat chicken filets with 1st tbsp olive oil and place in skillet
3. Brown chicken on one side, about 5-6 minutes, turn and brown on 2nd side. (Alternatively, chicken may be grilled on an outside grill or barbecue).

4. Using fork or tongs, remove chicken to a clean plate.
5. Add the tomatoes, olives to skillet with 2nd tbsp olive oil, stir and cook for 5 minutes.
6. Add baby spinach leaves, stir and cook for 2 more minutes.
7. Divide mixture and place half on each plate. Put one chicken filet on top of the mixture, and sprinkle with feta cheese to serve.

Nutrition Facts for Mediterranean Grilled Chicken with Spinach

Amount Per Serving

Calories 451.4

Sodium 648.8 mg

Total Fat 25.4 g

Potassium 669.7 mg

Saturated Fat 7.5 g

Total Carbohydrate 7.1 g

Polyunsaturated Fat 2.8 g

Dietary Fiber 1.6 g

Monounsaturated Fat 13.2 g

Sugars 4.6 g

Cholesterol 130.6 mg

Protein 44.1 g

Dinner Recipe #18 - Steamed Seafood Mix with Tomatoes and Pasta

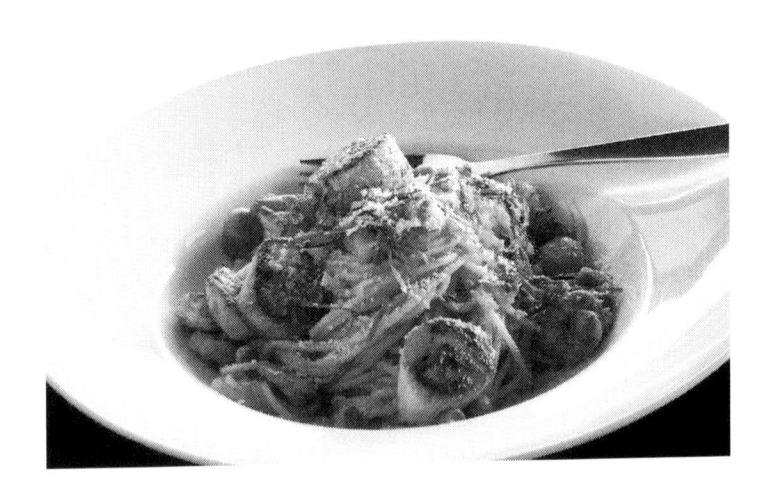

Servings: 2 adults
Preparation Time: 10 minutes
Cooking Time: 20 minutes

Follow **Dinner Recipe #14**, but instead of shrimp exclusively, use a variety of seafood ingredients. Buy what is at the market, as availability varies by season. For example, you can have a seafood selection that includes some or all of this assortment:

1 lb raw mix of scallops, small shrimp, scungilli (chopped conch), octopus, clams, mussels, as available. (If using large sea scallops, cut each in half)

Prepping and Cooking Directions: Same as for **Dinner Recipe #12,** but serve over pasta, simmered for 7-8 minutes until al-dente (cooked, with slight firmness, not soggy).

Nutrition Facts for Seafood with Tomatoes & Pasta

Amount Per Serving

Calories 465.7

Sodium 858.3 mg

Total Fat 13.9 g

Potassium 570.1 mg

Saturated Fat 2.2 g

Total Carbohydrate 26.9 g

Polyunsaturated Fat 2.8 g

Dietary Fiber 4.6 g

Monounsaturated Fat 7.2 g

Sugars 0.9 g

Cholesterol 351.3 mg

Protein 53.3 g

Conclusion

In reading this book, you have experienced self-discovery, and realized that your maturity is a good thing, but your health and wellbeing needs more attention. Now you are armed to take the personal initiative with your life. This book is the only guide you will need to get you there.

To summarize:

You are now ready to adopt a proactive lifestyle that really works, and is backed by science and experience. Your health involves more than trying to cope with being a middle age man; it requires a *personal lifestyle reinvention* to restore lost energy, become healthier, and feel better than you have in years. **This book is your personal roadmap** to slow the effects of aging, your personal step-by-step guide that combines scientific research and personal experience to optimize your diet and nutrition, improve your health, and strengthen you physically and emotionally, to manage your weight without counting calories.

As a man over 50, and concerned about your health and wellbeing, you are not alone. All men experience at least some of the physical and emotional changes and challenges that come with reaching 50 years of age, and the years that follow. You have a choice: to surrender to the inevitable signs and symptoms of aging, or to take charge of your health and your life, with the guidance and inspiration this book will provide.

It's common to be experiencing physical and emotional problems that arise when you are middle age. Do you think that your dietary practices may not be optimal for your health? Are you remembering when you kept in shape, and are wondering if it's possible to bring back the energy and vitality of when you were younger?

It's not too late to turn around what you thought were the inevitable downturns of health and fitness—both physical and mental. Starting now, you can begin to reverse the signs of aging, potentially increasing your longevity, and keeping you healthier and happier longer.

Reaching age 50 is a milestone to be proud of, but it's also a time to evaluate how you're doing and how it's going. Whether you're just hitting 50, or have gone beyond the half-century mark, the goal is to be in the best health and best shape you can be. But it's important to recognize and acknowledge that you've changed, and will continue to change as the years inevitably accumulate. Your shape is changing, and that lower gut is making its presence known. With the guidance this book provides, you are now ready to manage these changes, positively and effectively.

If you thought that a healthy diet would be difficult, you now know that it is easier than you think, with no need to limit your diet to bland and boring foods. You will discover new foods and eating practices that you can embrace with enthusiasm. Get ready to take realistic, achievable steps to prevent age-related health problems.

In closing, let me wish you every success in your new, energized, healthy lifestyle. If this book has met or exceeded your expectations, I hope you'll encourage your friends and mature contemporaries to read it.

I put a lot of effort to put this book together. A good rating on Amazon would be much appreciated, so that others will be encouraged to read it too. Your review is very important for me and for this book. I will be there to read it.

Warmest personal regards,

Michael Smith,

Boca Raton, Florida, 2020

Your Free Gift

To accelerate your journey towards optimum health **from today**

Go to link

[**bit.ly/mediterraneanshopping**](bit.ly/mediterraneanshopping)

to get a FREE PDF

MEDITERRANEAN DIET SHOPPING LIST with tips how often to eat certain foods

By joining my newsletter, you will be notified when my books are free on Amazon, so you can download them and not have to pay!

You will also be notified when I release a new book and be able to get it for a reduced price.

References

Addiction Campuses Editorial Team. (2019, September 30). How many drinks per week is too much? https://www.addictioncampuses.com/alcohol/how-many-drinks-is-too-much/

All images were retrieved from Pixabay.com and Unsplash.com.

Ambardekar, N. (2020, May 30). Guide to your immune system. *WebMD*. https://www.webmd.com/cold-and-flu/ss/slideshow-immune-system?ecd=wnl_spr_060820_PTID&ctr=wnl-spr-060820-PTID_nsl-Bodymodule_Position4&mb=MukfT6opS3AxbF5kSEwIong0WleHxvIqssh%40W36l9r4%3d

American Heart Association. (2020). Dietary fats. https://www.heart.org/en/healthy-living/healthy-eating/eat-smart/fats/dietary-fats

American Heart Association. (2019, May 24). Drinking red wine for heart health? Read this before you toast. https://www.heart.org/en/news/2019/05/

24/drinking-red-wine-for-heart-health-read-this-before-you-toast

Bank, S. (2020, February 6). The Obesity Code review: 10 things you need to know. *Diet spotlight.* https://www.dietspotlight.com/the-obesity-code-review/

Basaraba, S. (2020, March 22). Calorie requirement for seniors. *Verywell Fit.* https://www.verywellfit.com/calorie-requirements-for-older-people-2223969

Beauchesne, A. (2020, May 14). Plant-based diets and 3 types of arthritis: a look at the evidence. *Forks Over Knives.* https://www.forksoverknives.com/wellness/arthritis-plant-based-diets-scientific-evidence/#gs.7sir6c

Bhargava, H. (20202, March 26).Things that suppress your immune system. *WebMS.* https://www.webmd.com/cold-and-flu/ss/slideshow-how-you-suppress-immune-system?ecd=wnl_spr_061120&ctr=wnl-spr-061120_nsl-Bodymodule_Position6&mb=MukfT6opS3AxbF5kSEwIong0WleHxvIqssh%40W36l9r4%3d

Boyles, S. and Lloyd-Jones, D. (2006, February 6). How great is your heart attack risk at 50? *WebMD*. https://www.webmd.com/heart-disease/news/20060206/how-great-is-your-heart-risk-at-50#1

Campbell, T.C. and Esseltstyn, C. (2011). Forks Over Knives. https://www.forksoverknives.com/

Capritto, A. (2020, February 2). Water vs. Gatorade: Which is better to drink when you exercise? *CNET Health and Wellness*. https://www.cnet.com/health/water-vs-sports-drink-which-is-better-for-workout-hydration/

Carothers, J. (2018). 13 Tips to help men live happier, healthier and longer lives, *SLMA*. https://www.slma.cc/mens-health-month-13-tips-to-help-men-live-happier-healthier-and-longer-lives/

CDC. (2020). How much sleep do you need? https://www.cdc.gov/sleep/about_sleep/how_much_sleep.html

Cho, L. (2020, January 26). Heart disease: men vs. women. *Verywell Health*. https://www.verywellhealth.com/heart-disease-men-vs-women-4126017

Cleveland Clinic. (2020). Mens 'health: Lifestyle tips for men over 50 . https://my.clevelandclinic.org/health/articles/16422-mens-health-lifestyle-tips-for-men-over-age-50

Coleman, E. (2020). How much protein does meat have? *Live Strong*. https://www.livestrong.com/article/533434-how-much-protein-does-meat-have/

Cronkleton, E. (2020, April 1). The benefits of meditation walks. *Healthline*. https://www.healthline.com/health/walking-meditation?slot_pos=article_1&utm_source=Sailthru%20Email&utm_medium=Email&utm_campaign=generalhealth&utm_content=2020-06-04&apid=25264436

Doheny, C. (2012, November 30). Do older adults need vitamins, supplements? *WebMD*. https://www.webmd.com/healthy-aging/news/20121130/older-adults-vitamins-supplements#1

Edwards, T. (2018, January 16). Healthy weight loss = 80% nutrition + 20% exercise. *T. Colin Campbell Center for Nutrition Studies.*

https://nutritionstudies.org/healthy-weight-loss-80-nutrition-20-exercise/

Framingham Heart Study. (2020). Risk functions. *A project of Boston University & the National Heart, Lung, & Blood Institute.* https://framinghamheartstudy.org/

Fung, J. (2016). The Obesity Code: Unlocking the secrets of weight loss. *Greystone Books Ltd, Canada.* http://www.greystonebooks.com

Gomez, A. (2016, September 2). Is weight loss really 80% diet and 20% exercise? *Prevention.* https://www.prevention.com/weight-loss/a20474357/weight-loss-80-percent-diet-and-20-percent-exercise/

Green, S. (2017, July 28). Low testosterone, causes and symptoms. *Saga.* https://www.saga.co.uk/magazine/health-wellbeing/wellbeing/testosterone-levels-truth

Gunnars, K. (2020, April 6). 10 Evidence-basis benefits of green tea. *Healthline.* https://www.healthline.com/nutrition/top-10-evidence-based-health-benefits-of-green-tea?slot_pos=article_1&utm_source=Sailthru%20Email&utm_medium=Email&utm_c

ampaign=generalhealth&utm_content=2020-06-16&apid=25264436

Gunners, K. (2020, March 17). 6 Simple ways to lose belly fat, based on science. *Healthline.* https://www.healthline.com/nutrition/6-proven-ways-to-lose-belly-fat?slot_pos=article_1&utm_source=Sailthru%20Email&utm_medium=Email&utm_campaign=generalhealth&utm_content=2020-06-11&apid=25264436

Harvard Health Publishing. (2014). Health benefits linked to drinking tea. *Harvard Medical School.* https://www.health.harvard.edu/press_releases/health-benefits-linked-to-drinking-tea

Harvard T.H. Chan. (2020). The nutrition source. *School of Public Health.* https://www.hsph.harvard.edu/nutritionsource/

Hirsch, D. (2017). A medical review of the documentary Forks Over Knives. *David Z Hirsch.* https://davidzhirsch.wordpress.com/2017/08/27/a-medical-review-of-the-documentary-forks-over-knives/

Jennings, K-A. (2020, May 5). Collagen-What is it and what is it good for? *Healthline.* https://www.healthline.com/nutrition/collagen

Johnston, C. And Gass, C. (2006, May 30). Vinegar: medicinal uses and anti glycemic effect. *Medscape General Medicine.* https://www.ncbi.nlm.nih.gov/pmc/articles/PMC1785201/

Johns Hopkins (2020). FODMAP diet: what you need to know. *Johns Hopkins Medicine - Health.* https://www.hopkinsmedicine.org/health/wellness-and-prevention/fodmap-diet-what-you-need-to-know

Jong, N. (2017, September 12). 10 healthy reasons to drink coffee. *One Medical,* https://www.onemedical.com/blog/newsworthy/10-healthy-reasons-to-drink-coffee-2/

Kittridge, C. (2018, January 25). How much sleep to you really need? *Everyday Health.* https://www.everydayhealth.com/sleep/101/how-much-sleep-do-you-need.aspx

Klemm, S. (2020, May 21). Special nutrient needs of older adults. *Eat Right - Academy of Nutrition and Dietetics.*

https://www.eatright.org/health/wellness/healthy-aging/special-nutrient-needs-of-older-adults

Lehman, S. (2020, May 3). Potato nutrition facts and health benefits. *Very Well Fit.* https://www.verywellfit.com/are-potatoes-good-for-you-2506382

Link, R. (2018, March 19). Add vinegar to your diet. *Healthline.* https://www.healthline.com/nutrition/best-ways-to-burn-fat#section4

MacGill, M. (2017, November 13). Acid reflux: causes, treatments and symptoms. *Medical News Today.* https://www.medicalnewstoday.com/articles/146619

Mayo Clinic Staff. (2020). Belly fat in men: why weight loss matters. https://www.mayoclinic.org/healthy-lifestyle/mens-health/in-depth/belly-fat/art-20045685

Mayo Clinic Staff. (2020). Nutrition and health: alcohol use: weighing risks and benefits. https://www.mayoclinic.org/healthy-lifestyle/nutrition-and-healthy-eating/in-depth/alcohol/art-20044551

Mayo Clinic Staff. (2020). DASH diet: Healthy eating to lower your blood pressure. https://www.mayoclinic.org/healthy-lifestyle/nutrition-and-healthy-eating/in-depth/dash-diet/art-20048456

Men's Health. (2004, May 8). 50's - What changes and how to fix it. https://www.menshealth.com/health/a19526344/50s-what-changes-how-to-fix-it/

Men's Health Forum. (2014, April 8). Food FAQs. https://www.menshealthforum.org.uk/food-faqs

Men's Health Forum. (2015, June 18). Food supplements - do you need vitamins, minerals, or other extras? https://www.menshealthforum.org.uk/food-supplements

Men's Health Forum. (2015). Fitness FAQs. https://www.menshealthforum.org.uk/fitness-faqs

Mount Sinai Health System. (2020, June 1). Exercise levels can help doctors predict risk of heart disease and death among older adults. *News Wise*. https://www.newswise.com/articles/exercise-levels-can-help-doctors-predict-risk-of-heart-disease-and-death-among-older-adults

Nicolas, D. (2020). Diets for men over 50 . *Live Strong.* https://www.livestrong.com/article/216369-diets-for-men-over-50/

Ratini, M. (2018, November 30). Sudden health problems after 50. *WebMD.* https://www.webmd.com/healthy-aging/ss/slideshow-sudden-problems-after-50

Recipe of Health. (2020). Sports drinks results. http://recipeofhealth.com/nutrition-calories/search/calories-in-sports-drinks

Smith, V. (2020, June 4). I tried these 8 sleep tricks - here's what worked (and what didn't). *Get Pocket.* https://getpocket.com/explore/item/i-tried-these-8-sleep-tricks-here-s-what-worked-and-what-didn-t?utm_source=pocket-newtab

Stewart, J. (2019, December 13). 12 Simple ways for men to lose weight after 50. *Men's Health.* https://www.menshealth.com/weight-loss/a26555881/losing-weight-after-50/

Team Legion. (2020). 6 Amazing things that happen when you drink less alcohol. *Legion Athletics*. https://legionathletics.com/what-happens-when-you-stop-alcohol/

UCSF. (2020). Diabetes education online. https://dtc.ucsf.edu/types-of-diabetes/type1/understanding-type-1-diabetes/how-the-body-processes-sugar/controlling-blood-sugar/

USDA. (2020). Make better beverages. *Choose My Plate*. https://www.choosemyplate.gov/ten-tips-make-better-beverage-choices

US News & World Report. (2020). Best diets overall. https://health.usnews.com/best-diet/best-diets-overall

Wallace, R. And Yoder, K. (2019, April 25). 12 signs of low testosterone. *Healthline*. https://www.healthline.com/health/low-testosterone/warning-signs

WebMD. (2020). 13 tips to strengthen your immune system. https://www.webmd.com/diet/ss/slideshow-strengthen-immunity

WebMD. (2020). Guide to your immune system. https://www.webmd.com/cold-and-flu/ss/slideshow-immune-system?ecd=wnl_spr_060820_PTID&ctr=

wnl-spr-060820-PTID_nsl-Bodymodule_Position4&mb=MukfT6opS3AxbF5kSEwIong0WleHxvIqssh%40W36l9r4%3d

WebMD. (2020). Understanding osteoporosis-symptoms. https://www.webmd.com/osteoporosis/guide/understanding-osteoporosis-symptoms?ecd=wnl_hbn_060820&ctr=wnl-hbn-060820_nsl-Bodymodule_Position1&mb=MukfT6opS3AxbF5kSEwIong0WleHxvIqssh%40W36l9r4%3d

WebMD. (2020). Why are my joints so stiff? What can I do? https://www.webmd.com/rheumatoid-arthritis/ss/slideshow-stiff-joints?ecd=wnl_hbn_060820&ctr=wnl-hbn-060820_nsl-LeadModule_cta&mb=MukfT6opS3AxbF5kSEwIong0WleHxvIqssh%40W36l9r4%3d

WebMD. (2020). Health tips for men in their 60s and up. https://www.webmd.com/men/guide/simple-health-steps-men-60s-up

Weiler, L. (2018, September 4). Health advice men over 50 need to pay attention to. *Showbiz*

Cheat Sheet. https://www.cheatsheet.com/health-fitness/health-advice-men-over-50-need-to-pay-attention-to.html/

West, H. (2016, July 18). 18 Foods and drinks that are surprisingly high in sugar. *Healthline.* https://www.healthline.com/nutrition/18-surprising-foods-high-in-sugar

Printed in Great Britain
by Amazon